Antimicrobial Resistance and Antimicrobial Therapy of Clinically Relevant Bacteria

Antimicrobial Resistance and Antimicrobial Therapy of Clinically Relevant Bacteria

Guest Editors

Georgios Meletis
Lemonia Skoura
Efthymia Protonotariou

MDPI

Basel • Beijing • Wuhan • Barcelona • Belgrade • Novi Sad • Cluj • Manchester

Guest Editors
Georgios Meletis
Department of Microbiology
Aristotle University of Thessaloniki
Thessaloniki
Greece

Lemonia Skoura
AHEPA University Hospital
Aristotle University of Thessaloniki
Thessaloniki
Greece

Efthymia Protonotariou
AHEPA University Hospital
Aristotle University of Thessaloniki
Thessaloniki
Greece

Editorial Office
MDPI AG
Grosspeteranlage 5
4052 Basel, Switzerland

This is a reprint of the Special Issue, published open access by the journal *Antibiotics* (ISSN 2079-6382), freely accessible at: https://www.mdpi.com/journal/antibiotics/special_issues/clinical_bacteria.

For citation purposes, cite each article independently as indicated on the article page online and as indicated below:

Lastname, A.A.; Lastname, B.B. Article Title. *Journal Name* **Year**, *Volume Number*, Page Range.

ISBN 978-3-7258-6077-7 (Hbk)
ISBN 978-3-7258-6078-4 (PDF)
https://doi.org/10.3390/books978-3-7258-6078-4

Contents

About the Editors vii

Georgios Meletis, Lemonia Skoura and Efthymia Protonotariou
Antimicrobial Resistance and Antimicrobial Therapy of Clinically Relevant Bacteria
Reprinted from: *Antibiotics* **2024**, *13*, 691, https://doi.org/10.3390/antibiotics13080691 1

Ji-Fang Yu, Jin-Tian Xu, Ao Feng, Bao-Ling Qi, Jing Gu, Jiao-Yu Deng and Xian-En Zhang
Competition between H_4PteGlu and H_2PtePAS Confers *para*-Aminosalicylic Acid Resistance in *Mycobacterium tuberculosis*
Reprinted from: *Antibiotics* **2024**, *13*, 13, https://doi.org/10.3390/antibiotics13010013 4

Charalampos Zarras, Elias Iosifidis, Maria Simitsopoulou, Styliani Pappa, Angeliki Kontou, Emmanuel Roilides and Anna Papa
Neonatal Bloodstream Infection with Ceftazidime-Avibactam-Resistant bla_{KPC-2}-Producing *Klebsiella pneumoniae* Carrying bla_{VEB-25}
Reprinted from: *Antibiotics* **2023**, *12*, 1290, https://doi.org/10.3390/antibiotics12081290 17

Nouf Al-Rashed, Khalid M. Bindayna, Mohammad Shahid, Nermin Kamal Saeed, Abdullah Darwish, Ronni Mol Joji and Ali Al-Mahmeed
Prevalence of Carbapenemases in Carbapenem-Resistant *Acinetobacter baumannii* Isolates from the Kingdom of Bahrain
Reprinted from: *Antibiotics* **2023**, *12*, 1198, https://doi.org/10.3390/antibiotics12071198 28

Maria Sdougka, Maria Simitsopoulou, Elena Volakli, Asimina Violaki, Vivian Georgopoulou, Argiro Ftergioti, et al.
Evaluation of Five Host Inflammatory Biomarkers in Early Diagnosis of Ventilator-Associated Pneumonia in Critically Ill Children: A Prospective Single Center Cohort Study
Reprinted from: *Antibiotics* **2023**, *12*, 921, https://doi.org/10.3390/antibiotics12050921 38

Areti Tychala, Georgios Meletis, Paraskevi Mantzana, Angeliki Kassomenaki, Charikleia Katsanou, Aikaterini Daviti, et al.
Replacement of the Double Meropenem Disc Test with a Lateral Flow Assay for the Detection of Carbapenemase-Producing Enterobacterales and *Pseudomonas aeruginosa* in Clinical Laboratory Practice
Reprinted from: *Antibiotics* **2023**, *12*, 771, https://doi.org/10.3390/antibiotics12040771 52

Sonia Quddus, Zainab Liaqat, Sadiq Azam, Mahboob Ul Haq, Sajjad Ahmad, Metab Alharbi and Ibrar Khan
Identification of Efflux Pump Mutations in *Pseudomonas aeruginosa* from Clinical Samples
Reprinted from: *Antibiotics* **2023**, *12*, 486, https://doi.org/10.3390/antibiotics12030486 63

Paraskevi Mantzana, Efthymia Protonotariou, Angeliki Kassomenaki, Georgios Meletis, Areti Tychala, Eirini Keskilidou, et al.
In Vitro Synergistic Activity of Antimicrobial Combinations against Carbapenem- and Colistin-Resistant *Acinetobacter baumannii* and *Klebsiella pneumoniae*
Reprinted from: *Antibiotics* **2023**, *12*, 93, https://doi.org/10.3390/antibiotics12010093 80

Martin Zermeño-Ruiz, Itzia A. Rangel-Castañeda, Daniel Osmar Suárez-Rico, Leonardo Hernández-Hernández, Rafael Cortés-Zárate, José M. Hernández-Hernández, et al.
Curcumin Stimulates the Overexpression of Virulence Factors in *Salmonella enterica* Serovar Typhimurium: In Vitro and Animal Model Studies
Reprinted from: *Antibiotics* **2022**, *11*, 1230, https://doi.org/10.3390/antibiotics11091230 92

About the Editors

Georgios Meletis

Georgios Meletis obtained a degree in Medicine at the University of Bologna, Italy, a Master's degree in Medical Research Methodology at the Aristotle University of Thessaloniki, Greece, followed by a PhD in Microbiology at the same institution. He specializes in Medical Biopathology focusing on Microbiology. He is currently Associate Professor of Medical Biopathology-Microbiology at the Department of Microbiology, Medical School, Aristotle University of Thessaloniki.

Lemonia Skoura

Lemonia Skoura obtained her MD and PhD degree from the Medical School of Aristotle University of Thessaloniki. She specialized in Medical Microbiology and Clinical Microbiology and is currently a Professor of Medical Biopathology-Microbiology at Aristotle University and Head of the Medical Microbiology Laboratory of AHEPA University Hospital.

Efthymia Protonotariou

Efthymia Protonotariou graduated from the Medical School, Aristotle University of Thessaloniki, and obtained her PhD degree from Athens Medical School. She specialized in Medical Microbiology and Clinical Microbiology. She is currently Associate Professor of Medical Biopathology-Microbiology at Aristotle University at the Medical Microbiology Laboratory of AHEPA University Hospital.

antibiotics

MDPI

Editorial

Antimicrobial Resistance and Antimicrobial Therapy of Clinically Relevant Bacteria

Georgios Meletis *, Lemonia Skoura and Efthymia Protonotariou

Department of Microbiology, AHEPA University Hospital, School of Medicine, Aristotle University of Thessaloniki, S. Kiriakidi Str. 1, 54636 Thessaloniki, Greece; mollyskoura@gmail.com (L.S.); protonotariou@auth.gr (E.P.)
* Correspondence: meletisg@hotmail.com; Tel.: +30-697-428-2575

Antimicrobial resistance is a major public health problem, and the World Health Organization (WHO) has warned that the current antibiotic armamentarium is not sufficient to face future challenges. There are several obstacles to the antibiotic pipeline providing new compounds at a sufficient speed [1]. As a result, at present, few novel drugs reach clinical practice, with old, formerly abandoned antimicrobials increasingly used as last-resort treatment options instead [2]. At this pace, untreatable infections could emerge at a large scale, and the world may experience dramatic situations reminiscent of the pre-antibiotic era in some cases [3]. Already, clinicians in endemic areas routinely encounter patients with infections unresponsive to the available treatments, and laboratories often report multidrug-resistant (MDR) or even pan-drug-resistant (PDR) bacteria [4]. In this context, continuous monitoring of the epidemiology of the resistance mechanisms of clinically relevant bacteria, as well as knowledge regarding the treatment options, are of great interest to healthcare professionals. This Special Issue covers manuscript submissions that further our understanding of antimicrobial resistance in clinically relevant bacteria, suggest improved methods for detecting their underlying mechanisms and provide new insights into the treatment options. Submissions on alternative or new antimicrobial compounds and the in vitro susceptibility of relevant bacteria to such compounds were especially encouraged. Based on the comments and evaluations of the reviewers and editors, eight manuscripts were selected for publication, with each one providing a unique and valuable perspective pertaining to the topics of this Special Issue.

Para-Aminosalicylic acid (PAS) is an integral anti-tuberculosis drug which requires sequential activation by two Mycobacterial compounds. Previous studies have shown that specific mutations of the *thyA* gene cause PAS resistance in *Mycobacterium tuberculosis*, but the underlying mechanisms remained unclear. In the first article in this Special Issue, Yu et al. reveal how *thyA* mutations confer PAS resistance, outlining new findings on the folate metabolism of *M. tuberculosis*.

Ceftazidime–avibactam (CAZ/AVI) is an indispensable, potentially life-saving recent addition to the treatment options for non metallo-β-lactamase-producing Gram-negative pathogens, especially KPC-producing *Klebsiella pneumoniae*. Despite its relevance, however, there are no recommendations available for its use in neonates. In the second article in this issue, Zarras et al. report a Greek case of neonatal sepsis caused by CAZ/AVI-resistant KPC-2-encoding *K. pneumoniae*, which co-harbored the $bla_{\text{VEB-25}}$ gene.

Carbapenem-resistant *Acinetobacter baumannii* (CRAB) ranks high on the WHO global pathogen list and is widespread in many parts of the globe. Unfortunately, the epidemiologic situation of CRAB is poorly understood for certain countries, including Bahrain. Al-Rashed et al. shed light on this topic, demonstrating the prevalence of carbapenemases in CRAB isolated from four major hospitals within the Kingdom of Bahrain.

Due to the subjectivity of the clinical criteria and the low discriminative power of the diagnostic tests used, diagnosing ventilator-associated pneumonia (VAP) early remains a challenge. Therefore, novel biomarkers are urgently needed. In the fourth article in this issue, Sdougka et al. evaluated five host inflammatory biomarkers for the early diagnosis of VAP in critically ill children.

Promptly detecting carbapenemases in clinical and/or surveillance isolates recovered from healthcare settings such as hospital wards or ICUs is crucial for the timely implementation of infection control measures. In the fifth article in this issue, Tychala et al. evaluated the effectiveness and benefits of replacing the traditional phenotypic methods with a rapid immunochromatographic assay for Enterobacterales and *Pseudomonas aeruginosa*.

Efflux pumps represent an important bacterial mechanism conferring multi-drug resistance in Gram-negative bacteria; however, they have been less frequently investigated than enzymatic resistance determinants. In their study, Quddus et al. report intriguing efflux pump mutations in *P. aeruginosa* isolates from Pakistan.

Despite polymyxins commonly being used as a last-resort treatment for *A. baumannii* and *K. pneumoniae*, polymyxin resistance is on the rise worldwide. In an effort to diversify the treatment options for these stubborn sources of infection, Mantzana et al. assessed the in vitro synergistic activity of using specific antimicrobial combinations against carbapenem-resistant and colistin-resistant *A. baumannii* and *K. pneumoniae*.

The increasing resistance of *Salmonella* spp. to antimicrobials has galvanized the search for new alternatives, including natural compounds such as curcumin. In the final article in this Special Issue, Zermeño-Ruiz et al. aimed to verify the antibacterial activity of curcumin in relation to the growth rate, virulence and pathogenicity of *Salmonella enterica* serovar Typhimurium. Based on their results, the authors suggest reconsidering the indiscriminate use of curcumin in response to outbreaks of pathogenic Gram-negative bacteria.

Overall, the articles included in this Special Issue of Antibiotics offer new data on the antimicrobial resistance and epidemiology of MDR bacterial infections of key clinical importance, as well as suitable therapeutic options for their treatment. Hopefully, these contributions will both practically benefit the readership and stimulate further research in the field of antimicrobial resistance.

Conflicts of Interest: The authors declare no conflicts of interest.

List of Contributions:

1. Yu, J.-F.; Xu, J.-T.; Feng, A.; Qi, B.-L.; Gu, J.; Deng, J.-Y.; Zhang, X.-E. Competition between H_4PteGlu and H_2PtePAS Confers *para*-Aminosalicylic Acid Resistance in *Mycobacterium tuberculosis*. *Antibiotics* **2024**, *13*, 13. https://doi.org/10.3390/antibiotics13010013
2. Zarras, C.; Iosifidis, E.; Simitsopoulou, M.; Pappa, S.; Kontou, A.; Roilides, E.; Papa, A. Neonatal Bloodstream Infection with Ceftazidime-Avibactam-Resistant *bla*$_{KPC-2}$-Producing *Klebsiella pneumoniae* Carrying *bla*$_{VEB-25}$. *Antibiotics* **2023**, *12*, 1290. https://doi.org/10.3390/antibiotics12081290
3. Al-Rashed, N.; Bindayna, K.M.; Shahid, M.; Saeed, N.K.; Darwish, A.; Joji, R.M.; Al-Mahmeed, A. Prevalence of Carbapenemases in Carbapenem-Resistant *Acinetobacter baumannii* Isolates from the Kingdom of Bahrain. *Antibiotics* **2023**, *12*, 1198. https://doi.org/10.3390/antibiotics12071198
4. Sdougka, M.; Simitsopoulou, M.; Volakli, E.; Violaki, A.; Georgopoulou, V.; Ftergioti, A.; Roilides, E.; Iosifidis, E. Evaluation of Five Host Inflammatory Biomarkers in Early Diagnosis of Ventilator-Associated Pneumonia in Critically Ill Children: A Prospective Single Center Cohort Study. *Antibiotics* **2023**, *12*, 921. https://doi.org/10.3390/antibiotics12050921
5. Tychala, A.; Meletis, G.; Mantzana, P.; Kassomenaki, A.; Katsanou, C.; Daviti, A.; Kouroudi, L.; Skoura, L.; Protonotariou, E. Replacement of the Double Meropenem Disc Test with a Lateral Flow Assay for the Detection of Carbapenemase-Producing Enterobacterales and *Pseudomonas aeruginosa* in Clinical Laboratory Practice. *Antibiotics* **2023**, *12*, 771. https://doi.org/10.3390/antibiotics12040771
6. Quddus, S.; Liaqat, Z.; Azam, S.; Haq, M.U.; Ahmad, S.; Alharbi, M.; Khan, I. Identification of Efflux Pump Mutations in *Pseudomonas aeruginosa* from Clinical Samples. *Antibiotics* **2023**, *12*, 486. https://doi.org/10.3390/antibiotics12030486

7. Mantzana, P.; Protonotariou, E.; Kassomenaki, A.; Meletis, G.; Tychala, A.; Keskilidou, E.; Arhonti, M.; Katsanou, C.; Daviti, A.; Vasilaki, O.; et al. In Vitro Synergistic Activity of Antimicrobial Combinations against Carbapenem- and Colistin-Resistant *Acinetobacter baumannii* and *Klebsiella pneumoniae*. *Antibiotics* **2023**, *12*, 93. https://doi.org/10.3390/antibiotics12010093
8. Zermeño-Ruiz, M.; Rangel-Castañeda, I.A.; Suárez-Rico, D.O.; Hernández-Hernández, L.; Cortés-Zárate, R.; Hernández-Hernández, J.M.; Camargo-Hernández, G.; Castillo-Romero, A. Curcumin Stimulates the Overexpression of Virulence Factors in *Salmonella enterica* Serovar Typhimurium: In Vitro and Animal Model Studies. *Antibiotics* **2022**, *11*, 1230. https://doi.org/10.3390/antibiotics11091230

References

1. Theuretzbacher, U.; Baraldi, E.; Ciabuschi, F.; Callegari, S. Challenges and shortcomings of antibacterial discovery projects. *Clin. Microbiol. Infect.* **2023**, *29*, 610–615. [CrossRef] [PubMed]
2. Theuretzbacher, U.; Van Bambeke, F.; Cantón, R.; Giske, C.G.; Mouton, J.W.; Nation, R.L.; Paul, M.; Turnidge, J.D.; Kahlmeter, G. Reviving old antibiotics. *J. Antimicrob. Chemother.* **2015**, *70*, 2177–2181. [CrossRef]
3. Meletis, G. Carbapenem resistance: Overview of the problem and future perspectives. *Ther. Adv. Infect. Dis.* **2015**, *3*, 15–21. [CrossRef]
4. Ozma, M.A.; Abbasi, A.; Asgharzadeh, M.; Pagliano, P.; Guarino, A.; Köse, Ş.; Kafil, H.S. Antibiotic therapy for pan-drug-resistant infections. *Le Infez. Med.* **2022**, *30*, 525–531. [CrossRef]

antibiotics

Article

Competition between H_4PteGlu and H_2PtePAS Confers *para*-Aminosalicylic Acid Resistance in *Mycobacterium tuberculosis*

Ji-Fang Yu [1], Jin-Tian Xu [2,3], Ao Feng [2,3], Bao-Ling Qi [4], Jing Gu [2], Jiao-Yu Deng [2,*] and Xian-En Zhang [1,5,*]

1 Faculty of Synthetic Biology, Shenzhen Institute of Advanced Technology, Chinese Academy of Sciences, Shenzhen 518055, China
2 Wuhan Institute of Virology, Center for Biosafety Mega-Science, Chinese Academy of Sciences, Wuhan 430071, China
3 University of Chinese Academy of Sciences, Beijing 100049, China
4 Shanghai Metabolome Institute-Wuhan (SMI), Wuhan 430000, China
5 National Laboratory of Biomacromolecules, Institute of Biophysics, Chinese Academy of Sciences, Beijing 100101, China
* Correspondence: dengjy@wh.iov.cn (J.-Y.D.); zhangxe@ibp.ac.cn (X.-E.Z.)

Abstract: Tuberculosis remains a serious challenge to human health worldwide. *para*-Aminosalicylic acid (PAS) is an important anti-tuberculosis drug, which requires sequential activation by *Mycobacterium tuberculosis* (*M. tuberculosis*) dihydropteroate synthase and dihydrofolate synthase (DHFS, FolC). Previous studies showed that loss of function mutations of a thymidylate synthase coding gene *thyA* caused PAS resistance in *M. tuberculosis*, but the mechanism is unclear. Here we showed that deleting *thyA* in *M. tuberculosis* resulted in increased content of tetrahydrofolate (H_4PteGlu) in bacterial cells as they rely on the other thymidylate synthase ThyX to synthesize thymidylate, which produces H_4PteGlu during the process. Subsequently, data of in vitro enzymatic activity experiments showed that H_4PteGlu hinders PAS activation by competing with hydroxy dihydropteroate (H_2PtePAS) for FolC catalysis. Meanwhile, over-expressing *folC* in Δ*thyA* strain and a PAS resistant clinical isolate with known *thyA* mutation partially restored PAS sensitivity, which relieved the competition between H_4PteGlu and H_2PtePAS. Thus, loss of function mutations in *thyA* led to increased H_4PteGlu content in bacterial cells, which competed with H_2PtePAS for catalysis by FolC and hence hindered the activation of PAS, leading to decreased production of hydroxyl dihydrofolate (H_2PtePAS-Glu) and finally caused PAS resistance. On the other hand, functional deficiency of *thyA* in *M. tuberculosis* pushes the bacterium switch to an unidentified dihydrofolate reductase for H_4PteGlu biosynthesis, which might also contribute to the PAS resistance phenotype. Our study revealed how *thyA* mutations confer PAS resistance in *M. tuberculosis* and provided new insights into studies on the folate metabolism of the bacterium.

Keywords: *Mycobacterium tuberculosis*; *para*-aminosalicylic acid; tetrahydrofolate; *thyA*

1. Introduction

Tuberculosis (TB), caused by *M. tuberculosis*, is an ancient infectious disease. Recent data released by the World Health Organization show that around 10 million people fell in with the disease every year worldwide [1]. The increasing spread of drug-resistant *M. tuberculosis* makes TB treatment more difficult, and drug resistance has become one of the major challenges. The best way to solve the above problem is to introduce new anti-TB drugs. However, no new first-line drug has been introduced in clinical TB treatment for more than 50 years, since rifampicin [2]. Therefore, rational use of existing anti-tuberculosis drugs is necessary. In addition, researchers also have made efforts in using phages as an individual or supplementary therapy to treat *M. tuberculosis* infections [3].

Folate is an essential nutrient for all sorts of life. Bacteria need to synthesize folate de novo, but mammals are unable to synthesize it, which makes the bacterial de novo folate biosynthesis pathway an ideal target for developing new antibacterial drugs [4]. As is well known, dihydropteroate (H_2Pte) is synthesized by dihydropteroate synthetase (DHPS, FolP) using *para*-aminobenzoic acid (*p*ABA) and 7,8-dihydropterin pyrophosphate (H_2PtePP) as substrates, which is further converted into dihydrofolate (H_2PteGlu) by FolC (Figure 1) [5]. Dihydrofolate reductase (DHFR, DfrA or RibD) and thymidylate synthase (ThyA or ThyX) maintain the interconversion and balance between H_2PteGlu, H_4PteGlu and 5, 10-methylenetetrahydrofolate (5, 10-m-H_4PteGlu) (Figure 1). PAS was first used as a first-line anti-TB drug in 1946 [6], and is presently still used for treating multiple drug-resistant TB [7]. The mechanism of action of PAS had been gradually discovered over 70 years of clinical utilization. As a structural analogue of *p*ABA, PAS is firstly catalyzed by the FolP1 of *M. tuberculosis* to form H_2PtePAS, an analogue of H_2Pte. Subsequently, H_2PtePAS was further catalyzed by the FolC, yielding H_2PtePAS-Glu [5] (Figure 1). Ultimately, H_2PtePAS-Glu inhibited the activity of *M. tuberculosis* DfrA (Figure 1), resulting in bacterial growth inhibition and cell death [8].

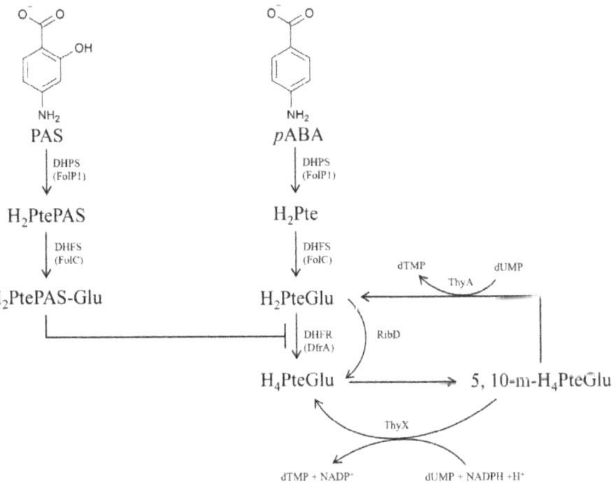

Figure 1. Schematic diagram of the mechanism of PAS action. PAS, *para*-aminosalicylic acid; *p*ABA, *para*-aminobenzoic acid; H_2PtePAS, hydroxy dihydropteroate; H_2Pte, dihydropteroate; H_2PtePAS-Glu, hydroxy dihydrofolate; H_2PteGlu, dihydrofolate; H_4PteGlu, tetrahydrofolate; 5, 10-m-H_4PteGlu, 5, 10-methylenetetrahydrofolate; DHPS/FolP1, dihydropteroate synthetase; DHFS/FolC, dihydrofolate synthase; DHFR/DfrA, dihydrofolate reductase; ThyA, thymidylate synthase; ThyX, thymidylate synthase; RibD, bifunctional diaminohydroxyphosphoribosylaminopyrimidine deaminase/5-amino-6-(5-phosphoribosylamino) uracil reductase.

Although the mechanism of PAS action has been elucidated, its mechanisms of resistance still await investigation. Until the present, confirmed molecular markers associated with PAS resistance in *M. tuberculosis* clinical isolates included mutations of *folC* [9–11], *thyA* [9,11–13], and *ribD* [8,9,11]. Among them, *folC* or *thyA* gene mutations were the main reasons for PAS resistance, accounting for two-thirds of the PAS resistant clinical isolates [9,11,14]. Molecular mechanisms of PAS resistance caused by *folC* and *ribD* mutations have been elucidated [8,10]. Our previous research showed that H_2Pte binding pocket variants of FolC failed to activate H_2PtePAS to H_2PtePAS-Glu, hindering the activation of PAS and hence conferring resistance to PAS [10]. On the other hand, *ribD* could serve as an alternative for DHFR, as mutations in the promoter region of the gene could cause over-expression of *ribD*, and thus lead to PAS resistance [8]. However, the molecular mechanism of PAS resistance caused by *thyA* mutations still remains unclear, though the association between *thyA* mutations and PAS resistance has been established for nearly two decades [13].

According to the data of epidemiological analysis, *thyA* mutations were identified in about 1/3 of the PAS resistant *M. tuberculosis* clinical isolates [9,11,12]. Thus, unravelling the mechanism of PAS resistance caused by *thyA* mutations will broaden our understanding of folate metabolism in *M. tuberculosis* and be useful for guiding the clinical administration of PAS. To elucidate how *thyA* mutations caused PAS resistance in *M. tuberculosis*, the *thyA* gene was deleted in H37Ra using the phage-mediated allelic exchange method, and a clinical PAS resistant isolate F461 harboring the *thyA* R235P mutation was selected [14]. Subsequently, the effect of *thyA* deletion on bacterial H_4PteGlu content was determined by UPLC-MS/MS. Then, the competition for catalysis of FolC between H_4PteGlu and H_2PtePAS was analyzed by in vitro enzymatic activity assays. Meanwhile, *folC* was over-expressed in the *thyA* deletion mutant and the selected PAS resistant clinical isolate, PAS susceptibilities of these two strains were tested. The level of FolC in ThyA deficiency strain was explored by RNA-seq and Western blot assays. The results are presented herein.

2. Results

2.1. *thyA* Deletion Leads to High Level PAS Resistance in *M. tuberculosis*

Considering the genetic complexity of clinical isolates, and also high similarity of mechanisms of PAS action and resistance between H37Ra and H37Rv [10], we constructed the *thyA* deletion strain in H37Ra to elucidate the molecular mechanism of how *thyA* mutations lead to PAS resistance in *M. tuberculosis*. H37Ra Δ*thyA* showed a significant growth defect (Figure S1), which is consistent with the observation in H37Rv Δ*thyA* [15]. Subsequently, the susceptibility to PAS was determined. The results showed that *thyA* deletion led to a hundreds of times increase in minimum inhibitory concentration (MIC) of PAS to *M. tuberculosis* (Table 1), which is consistent with clinical data [13]. After that, recombinant plasmids carrying *thyA* or *thyX* genes from *M. tuberculosis* H37Ra were used to transform H37Ra and H37Ra Δ*thyA*, respectively. Plasmid-borne expression of *thyA* restored PAS sensitivity of the *thyA* deletion strain, but that of *thyX* could not (Table 1). We noticed that over-expression of *thyA* and *thyX* both caused an eight times increase in PAS MIC (Table 1).

Table 1. *thyA* deletion confers PAS resistance in *M. tuberculosis* H37Ra.

Strains	MIC to PAS (μg mL^{-1})
H37Ra pMV261	0.04
H37Ra Δ*thyA* pMV261	10.24
H37Ra Δ*thyA* pMV261::*thyA*	0.32
H37Ra Δ*thyA* pMV261::*thyX*	10.24
H37Ra pMV261::*thyA*	0.32
H37Ra pMV261::*thyX*	0.32

2.2. *folC* Over-Expression Partially Restores PAS Sensitivity in *thyA* Functional Deficient Strains

Previous researches have confirmed that blocking the incorporation of PAS into folate synthesis pathway leads to high level resistance to PAS in *M. tuberculosis* [8,10]. To assess whether the high-level resistance to PAS of the *thyA* deletion strain was related to the efficiency of PAS incorporation, core genes *folP1*, *folC*, and *dfrA* of the folate biosynthesis pathway were over-expressed in H37Ra and H37Ra Δ*thyA*. The results showed that plasmid-borne expression of *folP1* and *folC* in H37Ra led to increased sensitivity to PAS, as demonstrated by the reduced MICs (four times for *folP1* over-expression and two times for *folC* over-expression) (Table 2). As the target for bio-activated PAS, *dfrA* over-expression increased the PAS MIC by thousands of times (Table 2). Over-expression of *folP1* in H37Ra Δ*thyA* also led to a four-times decrease in PAS MIC, which was consistent with that in H37Ra (Table 2). However, over-expressing *folC* in H37Ra Δ*thyA* led to a 16-times decrease in PAS MIC, and over-expressing *dfrA* in H37Ra Δ*thyA* did not change the PAS MIC (Table 2). To further prove that over-expressing *folC* could reverse the high-level PAS resistance phenotype in *thyA* functional deficient strains, *folC* was over-expressed in the

PAS resistant clinical isolate harboring the *thyA* R235P mutation. As shown in Table 2, *folC* over-expression also led to a 10-times decrease in PAS MIC in the clinical isolate.

Table 2. Over-expression of *folC* gene reverses the PAS resistance phenotype.

Strains	MIC to PAS (μg mL^{-1})
H37Ra pMV261	0.04
H37Ra pMV261::*folP1*	0.01
H37Ra pMV261::*folC*	0.02
H37Ra pMV261::*dfrA*	81.92
H37Ra Δ*thyA* pMV261	10.24
H37Ra Δ*thyA* pMV261::*folP1*	2.56
H37Ra Δ*thyA* pMV261::*folC*	0.64
H37Ra Δ*thyA* pMV261::*dfrA*	10.24
F461 *	500
F461 pMV261::*folC*	50

* Clinically isolated PAS resistant strain with *thyA* R235P mutation.

2.3. The Expression Level of folC Gene and FolC Protein Remain Unchanged in H37Ra ΔthyA

To further explore the role of *folC* in PAS resistance caused by ThyA functional deficiency, we detected the expression level of *folC* in wild-type and *thyA* deletion strain. Western blot assay was performed to compare the expression level of FolC between wild-type and *thyA* deletion strain, and the results showed that the FolC expression level was not significantly changed in the *thyA* deletion strain (Figure 2A,B). Meanwhile, RNA-seq data also showed that the expression level of *folC* was not significantly changed in the *thyA* deletion strain (Figure 2C).

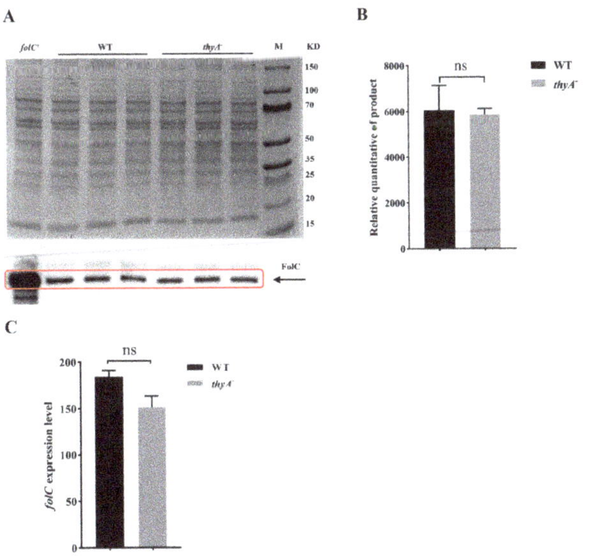

Figure 2. The expression of *folC* remains unchanged in ThyA functional deficient strain. (**A**) Comparison of the expressional level of FolC during the exponential phase in H37Ra (WT) and H37Ra Δ*thyA* (*thyA*$^{-}$) by Western blot assay. Upper part: Total protein was normalized to 25 μg of each strain, then electrophoresed by SDS-PAGE and stained by Coomassie brilliant blue. Lower part: Western blot analysis of total protein immunoblotted with rabbit FolC polyclonal antibody. Experiments were repeated at least three times, and were performed three biological replicates each time. (**B**) Relative quantitative of FolC product by Western blot assay. ns, no significance. (**C**) Comparison of the transcriptional level of the gene *folC* during the exponential phase in H37Ra (WT) and H37Ra Δ*thyA* (*thyA*$^{-}$) by RNA-seq. ns, no significance.

2.4. thyA Deletion Leads to Increased H_4PteGlu Content in Bacterial Cells

There are two types of thymidylate synthase, ThyA and ThyX, in *M. tuberculosis* [15], and the thymidylate synthase function is mainly performed by ThyA. ThyA uses 5, 10-m-H_4PteGlu as methyl donor to generate H_2PteGlu and maintain the balance of folate metabolism (Figure 1) [15,16], and ThyX uses 5, 10-m-H_4PteGlu as methyl donor to generate H_4PteGlu (Figure 1) [16,17]. After the loss of ThyA function, the bacterium relies on ThyX for synthesizing thymidylate [15]. Thus, we speculated that the H_4PteGlu content would increase in ThyA deficient strains. As expected, we observed an obvious increase in H_4PteGlu content in the *thyA* deletion strain compared to the wild-type strain (Figure 3).

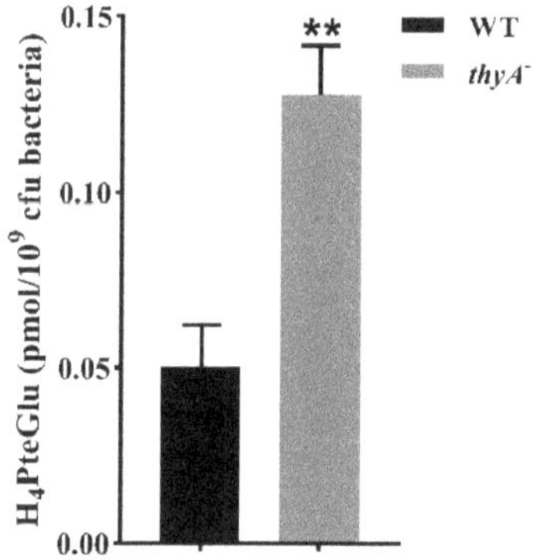

Figure 3. The quantitative detection of H_4PteGlu by UPLC-MS/MS in *thyA* deletion strain. Cell-associated H_4PteGlu was extracted from H37Ra (WT) and H37Ra Δ*thyA* (*thyA*$^-$). The experiments were performed using six biological replicates. *p*-values (*p*) were calculated using *t*-tests. ** $p < 0.01$.

2.5. Comparison of Catalytic Efficiency of FolC on H_2Pte, H_4PteGlu and H_2PtePAS

FolC was demonstrated to be a bifunctional enzyme in *Escherichia coli* (*E. coli*) which not only converted H_2Pte into H_2PteGlu, but also added glutamic acid tail to H_4PteGlu [18,19]. Therefore, we speculated that H_4PteGlu would also compete with H_2PtePAS for catalysis activity of FolC in *M. tuberculosis*, thus hindering the activation process of PAS. To test this speculation, catalytic efficiency of FolC on H_2Pte, H_4PteGlu, and H_2PtePAS was compared. The results showed that, under the same reaction conditions, FolC could convert about 85% H_2Pte and 50% H_4PteGlu, but only about 12% H_2PtePAS (Figure 4).

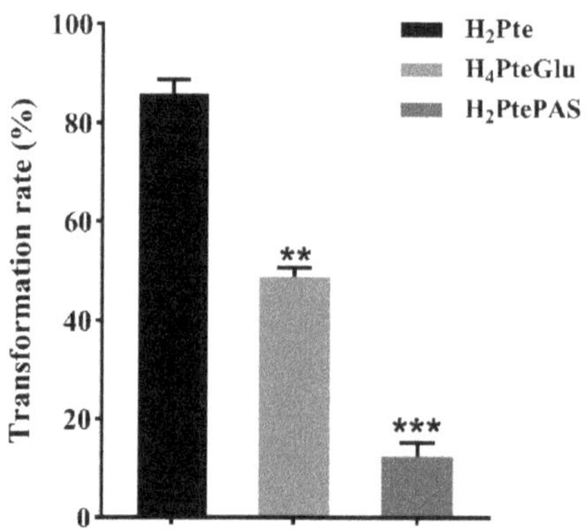

Figure 4. Catalytic utilization of H_2Pte, H_4PteGlu, and H_2PtePAS by DHFS. The experiments were performed using three biological replicates. *p*-values (*p*) were calculated using *t*-tests. ** $p < 0.01$, *** $p < 0.001$.

2.6. H_4PteGlu Hinders the Activation of PAS by FolC

To further demonstrate whether H_4PteGlu could hinder the activation of PAS by FolC, H_2PtePAS was synthesized by purified recombinant FolP1 using H_2PtePP and PAS as substrates [10]. H_2PtePAS was analyzed by UPLC-MS/MS (Figure 5A, Supplementary Table S1). FolC catalytic activity was analyzed using H_2PtePAS instead of H_2Pte as a substrate. Consistent with previous reports [5,10], FolC could catalyze the ligation of L-glutamic acid to H_2PtePAS generating H_2PtePAS-Glu, which was confirmed by HPLC-MS/MS (Figure 5B, Supplementary Table S1). We then sought to understand the effect of H_4PteGlu on H_2PtePAS activation by FolC, and different concentrations (10 μM and 50 μM) of H_4PteGlu were added into the FolC reaction mixture using H_2PtePAS as substrate. As shown in Figure 5C, when H_4PteGlu was added into the reaction mixture, the catalytic efficiency of FolC for H_2PtePAS decreased remarkably.

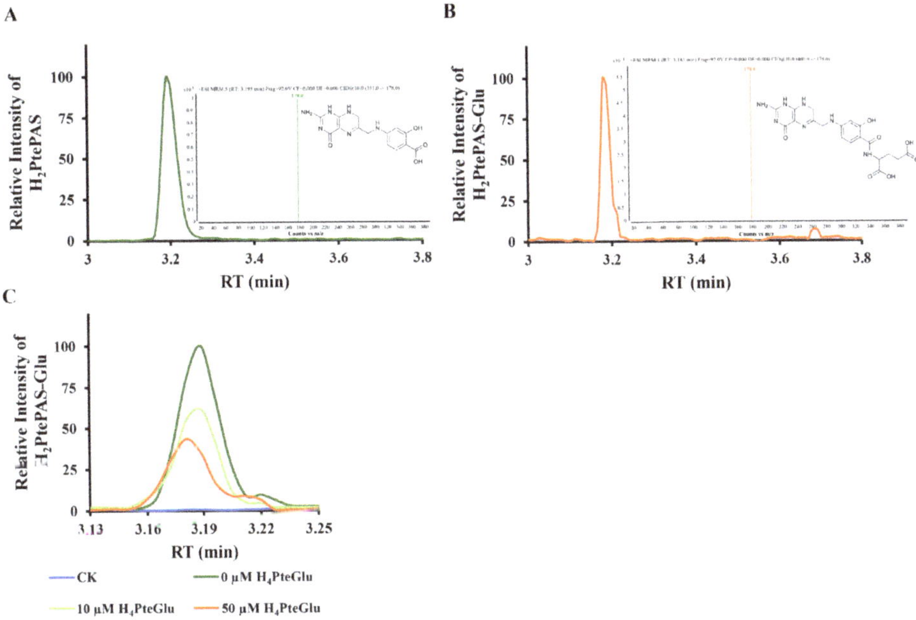

Figure 5. H_4PteGlu hinders the activation of PAS. (**A**) H_2PtePAS was identified based on HPLC-MS/MS. Retention time 3.193 min, ion channel 331.0 -> 178.0. (**B**) H_2PtePAS-Glu was identified based on HPLC-MS/MS. Retention time 3.181 min, ion channel 460.0 -> 178.0. (**C**) Extracted ion chromatograms of H_2PtePAS-Glu showing H_4PteGlu reduced the catalytic efficiency of FolC on H_2PtePAS.

3. Discussion

Folates, especially derivatives of H_4PteGlu, are one carbon carriers required by the biosynthesis of purines, thymidylate, methionine, serine, and glycine, thus making them essential for all sorts of lives [20,21]. Bacteria must synthesize these essential cofactors *de novo*, while mammal can intake them from their diet [4]. This difference makes the bacterial *de novo* folate biosynthesis pathway an ideal target for developing new antibacterial drugs [4]. Although thousands of folates antagonists have been designed for folate biosynthesis pathway heretofore, PAS is the only one used for TB treatment with a unique mode of action only observed in *M. tuberculosis* complex. Thus, better understanding the mechanisms of PAS resistance in *M. tuberculosis* will benefit the development of new antifolates against this bacterium.

As the first molecular marker for PAS resistance in *M. tuberculosis* clinical isolates, *thyA* gene mutations have been identified for nearly two decades [13], but the molecular mechanism of how these mutations lead to PAS resistance remains unknown. Ten years later, when probing the molecular mechanism of PAS resistance caused by *folC* mutation [10], we noticed that though FolC could also catalyze the conversion of H_2PtePAS to H_2PtePAS-Glu, but the catalytic efficiency was much lower than that of the natural substrate H_2Pte, implying that the bio-activation process of PAS might be vulnerable to interference of natural metabolite of folate biosynthesis. Indeed, exogenous H_2Pte made *M. tuberculosis* more resistant to PAS [10]. Previous studies have showed that FolC could not only convert H_2Pte into H_2PteGlu, but also add glutamic acid tail to H_4PteGlu in *E. coli* [18,19]. In this study, we found that *M. tuberculosis* FolC is also bifunctional. In addition, its catalytic efficiency for H_2PtePAS is remarkably lower than that for H_4PteGlu (Figure 4), implying intracellular H_4PteGlu may interfere the activation of PAS by FolC. As expected, the in vitro biochemical experiments showed that H_4PteGlu hinders the conversion of H_2PtePAS to H_2PtePAS-Glu in a concentration-dependent manner (Figure 5C). Since *M. tuberculosis* is not able to intake exogenous H_4PteGlu, it is not possible to test the effect of exogenous H_4PteGlu on PAS susceptibility. Alternatively, we compared the H_4PteGlu content between H37Ra and the *thyA* deletion mutant, and found that the H_4PteGlu content in the *thyA* deletion mutant was significantly higher than that of the wild-type strain (Figure 3). This is not surprising since the bacterium has to solely rely on ThyX to synthesize thymidylate in the absence of ThyA, and utilization of the former yields H_4PteGlu. Since the expression level of FolC remained unchanged in the *thyA* deletion mutant, increased H_4PteGlu content could hinder the conversion of H_2PtePAS since they compete for the same protein. Correspondingly, this competition could be mitigated by over-expression of the target protein FolC. As expected, over-expression of *folC* could reverse the PAS resistance phenotype caused by *thyA* deletion or clinical *thyA* R235P mutation (Table 2). We noticed that the PAS resistance phenotype caused by *thyA* deletion or mutation could only be partially restored by *folC* over-expression, suggesting the existence of other mechanisms for PAS resistance caused by functional deficiency of ThyA.

When assessing whether the resistance to PAS of the *thyA* deletion mutant was related to the efficiency of PAS activation, we over-expressed *folP1*, *folC*, and *dfrA* in H37Ra and H37Ra Δ*thyA*. To our surprise, over-expression of *dfrA* in the *thyA* deletion mutant did not affect the susceptibility to PAS (Table 2), suggesting either the lack of DfrA protein or loss of function of DfrA in the *thyA* deletion mutant. Previous works also showed that *thyA* and *dfrA* double deletion mutants had been identified in *M. tuberculosis* clinical isolates from different countries [11,22]. Thus, in the absence of *thyA*, *M. tuberculosis* discards the commonly used DHFR Rv2763c (DfrA), and switches to another alternative to synthesize H_4PteGlu. Although RibD was shown to be an alternative DHFR in *M. tuberculosis*, previous research revealed that RibD could only replace DfrA when it was highly over-expressed in a multi-copy plasmid [8], suggesting that the dihydrofolate reductase activity of RibD is quite low, which was confirmed by subsequent biochemical analysis [23]. Zheng et al. found that mutations in the promoter region of *ribD* could cause over-expression of *ribD* [8]. To determine whether RibD is the alternative DHFR in the absence of ThyA in *M. tuberculosis*, we further analyzed genome sequences of isolates with frameshift or deletion mutations in *thyA* or *dfrA* genes from previous studies and NCBI database. The results showed that there was no mutation in either the promoter region (300 bp upstream start codon) or the coding sequence (CDS) of the *ribD* gene in ThyA or DfrA deficient clinical isolates (Supplementary Table S2). Moreover, our RNA-seq data also showed that the expression level of *ribD* remained unchanged in the *thyA* deletion mutant (Figure S2). Therefore, RibD is not the alternative DHFR in the absence of ThyA. What the alternative DHFR is in the absence of ThyA requires further investigation. It will be important to test if the alternative DHFR would be more resistant to the inhibition of H_2PtePAS-Glu, since over-expressing *folC* could only partially restore PAS sensitivity to the *thyA* deletion mutant.

Previous studies already showed that the $C^{-16}T$ mutation in the upstream regulatory region of *thyX* could lead to increased expression of *thyX* and PAS resistance in *M. tuberculosis* [24,25]. Thus, it is not surprising to see that over-expressing *thyX* led to PAS resistance in H37Ra. The fact that over-expressing *thyX* in the *thyA* deletion mutant did not affect PAS susceptibility of the latter indicated that over-expressing *thyX* and deleting *thyA* in *Mtb* might share the same mechanism of PAS resistance. In addition, over-expressing *thyA* in H37Ra also led to low level PAS resistance. Considering the role of ThyA in folate salvage, we speculated that the intracellular H_2PteGlu content might be increased when over-expressing *thyA*; this would in turn reduce the demand for dihydrofolate biosynthesis through FolC. Previous studies showed that FolC was critical for the bio-activation of PAS, and decreased FolC enzymatic activity caused PAS resistance [8,10].

In conclusion, our results showed that functional deficiency of ThyA led to increased H_4PteGlu content of the bacterial cells, which competed with H_2PtePAS for FolC catalysis, thus hindered the activation of PAS and conferred PAS resistance in *M. tuberculosis*. Meanwhile, our study also suggested that *M. tuberculosis* could switch from Rv2763c to a yet unknown alternative DHFR in the absence of *thyA*, and further investigation is required to identify the protein and elucidate its role on PAS resistance caused by ThyA functional deficiency. Our study broadens the understanding of folate metabolism in *M. tuberculosis* and might be useful for guiding the clinical administration of PAS.

4. Materials and Methods

4.1. Bacterial Strains, Plasmids, and Growth Conditions

Clinical isolate F461, *M. tuberculosis* H37Ra and its derivative strains were cultured at 37 °C in 7H9 broth (Difco, St. Louis, MO, USA) supplemented with 10% (*v*/*v*) oleic acid-albumin-dextrose-catalase (OADC, Difco), 0.5% (*v*/*v*) glycerol, and 0.05% (*v*/*v*) Tween 80 (Sigma-Aldrich, St. Louis, MO, USA), or on 7H10 agar medium (Difco) supplemented with 10% (*v*/*v*) OADC and 0.5% (*v*/*v*) glycerol. *Mycobacterium smegmatis* mc^2155 was grown in Middlebrook 7H9 medium or 7H10 agar medium. *E. coli* strains HB101 and BL21 (DE3) were cultured in Luria-Bertani (LB) medium (Difco), or on LB agar plates at 37 °C. Plasmids pMAL-c2X (New England BioLabs, Beverly, MA, USA), pET-28a (Novagen, Madison, WI, USA), and pMV261 were used for the construction of expression plasmids. All bacteria strains, plasmids, and primers used in this study are described in detail in Supplementary Table S3.

4.2. Antibiotics and Chemicals

These concentrations of antibiotics (75 μg mL^{-1} and 150 μg mL^{-1} hygromycin (Sigma-Aldrich), 25 μg mL^{-1} and 100 μg mL^{-1} Kanamycin (MD Bio, Inc., Qingdao, China), and 150 μg mL^{-1} ampicillin (MD Bio, Inc.)) were used to culture bacteria, unless otherwise indicated. H_2Pte and H_4PteGlu were purchased from Schircks Laboratories. PAS (Sigma-Aldrich) was used at indicated concentrations.

4.3. Genetic Manipulation of Mycobacterial Strains

folC, *thyA*, *thyX*, *dfrA*, and *folP1* were amplified from wild-type *M. tuberculosis* H37Ra genomic DNA using PCR with the primers (Supplementary Table S3). The purified amplicon was digested and ligated to pMV261, generating pMV261-*folC*, pMV261-*thyA*, pMV261-*dfrA*, pMV261-*folP1*, and pMV261-*thyX*. *M. tuberculosis* strain was transformed with sequence-confirmed pMV261 recombinant plasmid, then plated on 7H10 medium containing 25 μg mL^{-1} kanamycin. After 3 weeks of incubation at 37 °C, single colonies were purified and liquid cultures were prepared for the extraction of genomic DNA and determination of PAS MICs, separately. The presence of pMV261 recombinant plasmid was verified by PCR amplification using primers specific for pMV261-JDFP and pMV261-JDRP (Supplementary Table S3).

A modified strategy for phage-mediated allelic exchange [26] was used to construct *M. tuberculosis* H37Ra Δ*thyA* mutant. Briefly, the native copy of *thyA* was deleted by specialized transduction using phAE159 containing a hygromycin resistance cassette. All primers used are listed in Supplementary Table S3.

4.4. Purification of Recombinant FolP1 and FolC

FolP1 and FolC proteins were purified as previously reported [10]. Briefly, *folP1* and *folC* were amplified from *M. tuberculosis* H37Ra genomic DNA using specific primers (Supplementary Table S3) and separately cloned into pET28a to yield pET28a::*folP1* to introduce an N-terminal hexa-histidine tag and into pMAL-c2X to yield pMAL-c2X::*folC* to introduce an N-terminal maltose-binding protein (MBP) tag linked with a factor Xa cleavage site. The sequence-confirmed recombinant plasmids were transformed into *E. coli* BL21 (DE3). The cells were grown at 37 °C in LB broth containing 150 μg mL^{-1} ampicillin or 100 μg mL^{-1} kanamycin to an OD_{600} of ~0.6. Isopropyl-β-D-thiogalactopyranoside (IPTG, Acmec, China) was added to 0.25 mM, then the cells were incubated further at 16 °C for 20 h. The bacterial cells were harvested by centrifugation, disrupted by sonication, and clarified by centrifugation.

Recombinant FolP1 protein was purified over prewashed nickel–nitrilotriacetic acid HisTrap HP affinity resin (GE Healthcare, Little Chalfont, Buckinghamshire, UK). Non-specifically bound protein was removed by washing the resin with 50 mM Tris-HCl, 0.5 M NaCl, and 60 mM imidazole (pH 8.0). Recombinant FolP1 was eluted with 50 mM Tris-HCl, 0.5 M NaCl, and 400 mM imidazole (pH 8.0), and analyzed by SDS-PAGE.

Recombinant FolC proteins were first purified over an amylose resin column (New England BioLabs). The FolC protein obtained from the first purification contains MBP tag. To remove the MBP tag, the purified samples were incubated with factor Xa at 4 °C overnight in reaction buffer (20 mM HEPES (pH 8.0), 100 mM NaCl, 2 mM $CaCl_2$, and 10% glycerol). Then, the cleavage mixtures were dialyzed against 50 mM phosphate buffer (pH 8.0). The samples were loaded on a HiTrap DEAE FF column (GE Healthcare), and a step gradient from 50 mM to 1 M NaCl in phosphate buffer was applied to elute FolC. The fractions were then analyzed by SDS-PAGE. Recombinant FolC was eluted with 300 mM NaCl.

4.5. Western Blot Assay

The H37Ra and H37Ra Δ*thyA* strains were cultured at 37 °C in 10 mL of 7H9 medium and harvested at logarithmic phase by centrifugation. For Western blot analysis, bacterial cells were resuspended in phosphate buffer saline (PBS, pH 7.0), then lysed using zirconium beads. Protein samples acquired from the supernatant after centrifugation. The protein concentration of the supernatant was determined using the NanoDrop2000 (Thermo, Waltham, MA, USA). Then, the protein samples were separated by SDS-PAGE and immediately transferred to a polyvinylidene difluoride membrane (Merck Millipore, Darmstadt, Germany) by a Bio-Rad SD device (Bio-Rad Laboratories, Hercules, CA, USA) at 15 V for 30 min. Finally, the proteins were probed with rabbit FolC polyclonal antibody (ABclonal biotechnology, Wuhan, China, Cat. No. WG-00133D).

4.6. RNA-Seq Analysis

Mycobacterial strains were grown in 7H9 to mid logarithmic phase and were collected by centrifugation. Total RNA was extracted using RNeasy mini kit (Qiagen, Hilden, Germany). Library constructions were prepared using TruSeq Stranded Total RNA Sample Preparation kit (Illumina, San Diego, CA, USA), and RNA sequencing was conducted on Illumina NovaSeq6000 at Beijing Novogene Corporation. The insert size conformation of purified libraries was validated by an Agilent 2100 bioanalyzer (Agilent Technologies, Santa Clara, CA, USA). Bowtie2 was used to map the cleaned reads to the M. tuberculosis H37Ra genome acquired from the National Center for Biotechnology Information (NCBI) (https://www.ncbi.nlm.nih.gov/nuccore/CP000611.1) (Accessed on 25 May 2023). Then, HTSeqv0.6.1 was run with a reference annotation to generate fragments per kilobase of exon model per million mapped reads values for estimation of fold changes. Three biological replicates were used in RNA-seq and the *p*- and q-values were calculated. The differentially expressed genes were selected using the following filter criteria: q-value < 0.005 and |log2 (fold change)| > 1. Raw RNA sequencing data have been deposited at NCBI Sequence Read Archive, Accession PRJNA1005084.

4.7. In Vitro Enzymatic Activity Assays

The dihydrofolate synthase activities of FolC using H_2Pte, H_2PtePAS, and H_4PteGlu as substrates were measured and H_2PtePAS was enzymatically synthesized as previously described [5,10]. Briefly, the reaction mixture contained 1.2 μM FolP1, 40 mM Tris-20 mM glycine (pH 9.5), 5 mM $MgCl_2$, 1 mM DTT, 200 mM NaCl, appropriate amounts of 6-hydroxymethyl-7,8-pterin pyrophosphate (H_2PtePP), and 250 μM PAS. The reaction mixture was incubated at 37 °C until no increment of H_2PtePAS accumulation was detected by UPLC-MS/MS. FolP1 was removed by passing through a 10-kDa Microcon centrifugal filter, and 325 μL of the remaining reaction mixture was used as a substrate for FolC. The FolC reaction mixture contained 0.5 μM FolC protein, 2.5 mM ATP, and 0.5 mM L-glutamate in 100 mM Tris-50 mM glycine (pH 9.5), 10 mM $MgCl_2$, 5 mM DTT, 100 mM KCl, 50 mM NaCl, 10% glycerol, appropriate amounts H_2PtePAS, and the presence/absence of H_4PteGlu. The mixture was incubated at 37 °C for 15 min. H_2Pte, H_2PtePAS, and H_4PteGlu were identified by UPLC-MS/MS. UPLC column was Waters ACQUITY UPLC HSS T3 Column (2.1 × 100 mm, 1.8 μm particles) using a flow rate of 0.4 mL/min at 40 °C during a 6 min gradient (0–1 min from 2% B to 1% B, 1–3.5 min from 1% B to 50% B, 3.5–3.8 min from 50% B to 95% B, 3.8–6 min 95% B), while using the solvents A (water containing 20 mM ammonium acetate) and B (methanol). Electrospray ionization was performed using the positive ion mode, the pressure of the nebulizer was 30 psi, the dry gas temperature was 325 °C with a flow rate of 11 L/min, the sheath gas temperature was 350 °C with a flow rate of 10 L/min, and the capillary was set at 4000 V. Multiple reaction monitoring (MRM) was used for the quantification of screening fragment ions. Peak determination and peak area integration were performed using Mass Hunter Workstation software (Agilent, Version B.08.00). *p*-values (*p*) were calculated using *t*-tests. The graphs for the transformation rate of H_2Pte, H_4PteGlu, and H_2PtePAS were prepared using GraphPad Prism.

4.8. Drug Susceptibility Testing

Mycobacterial cells were cultured to mid-log phase (OD_{600}: 0.5–1.0) and diluted to about 10^5 cfu mL^{-1} using 10-fold serial dilutions in fresh 7H9 medium with or without 10% OADC. Then, bacterial cells were plated on 7H10 agar solid plates containing various concentrations of PAS (0, 0.00125, 0.0025, 0.005, 0.01, 0.02, 0.04, 0.08, 0.16, 0.32, 0.64, 1.28, 2.56, 5.12, 10.24, 20.48, 40.96, and 81.92 μg mL^{-1}). PAS was purchased from Sigma-Aldrich and solubilized according to the manufacture's recommendations. Plates were then incubated at 37 °C for 21 days. The MIC was defined as the lowest concentration of antibiotics required to inhibit 99% of CFUs after this culture period. The MICs were performed through two technical repetitions using three biological replicates. All of the bacteria strains used are listed in Supplementary Table S3.

4.9. Determination of H_4PteGlu Content In Vivo

Bacteria samples (~5 × 10^9 cfu) were re-suspended in 0.4 mL pre-cooled 20 mM HEPES (containing 2% vitamin C and 1% dithiothreitol, pH 7.0) and subjected to three liquid nitrogen freeze–thaw cycles and zirconia bead grinding before sonication in an ice bath for 15 cycles (1 min pulse followed by 1 min pause). The above extraction procedure was repeated three times. The mixture was then centrifuged for 10 min at 12,000× *g* at 4 °C, and each supernatant was filtered using a 0.22 μm membrane filter before UPLC-MS/MS analysis. The samples were detected as above with some changes. Briefly, the samples (5 μL) were individually injected on an UPLC column (Agilent ZORBAX Eclipse Plus C_{18} column, 2.1 × 100 mm, 1.8 μm particles) using a flow rate of 0.4 mL/min at 50 °C using the solvents A (water containing 0.1% (*v*/*v*) formic acid) and B (methanol containing 0.1%

(v/v) formic acid). The bacterial biomasses of the individual samples were determined by colony counting method. All data obtained by metabolomics were averaged from the independent sextuplicates. p-values (p) were calculated using t-tests. The graphs for the determination of H_4PteGlu in vivo were prepared using GraphPad Prism.

4.10. Comparative Analysis of Variants in M. tuberculosis Genomes

M. tuberculosis clinical isolates with complete or partial deletion of *thyA* or *dfrA* were extensively collected from previous studies [11,22,27] and the NCBI database (https://www.ncbi.nlm.nih.gov/genome/browse#!/prokaryotes/mycobacterium%20tuberculosis) (Accessed on 7 December 2022). A total of 31 *M. tuberculosis* genomes from clinical isolates were obtained, and the mutations in the promoter region (300 bp upstream start codon) or the CDS of *ribD* were analyzed in these isolates (Supplemental Table S2). All of the raw reads were available. The acquired reads were subjected to quality assessment using FastQC v.0.11.9. Subsequently, low-quality sequences were removed and trimmed using fastp. Reads shorter than 50 bp were discarded, the last 10 bp were trimmed, and bases with an average quality below 25 were removed using a sliding window of 20 bp. Finally, variant calling against the *M. tuberculosis* H37Rv (NC_000962.3) genome was performed using the Snippy pipeline.

4.11. Statistical Analysis

GraphPad Prism 8.0.1 was used to analyze all experimental data, adopting the two-tailed unpaired t-test method. Mean ± standard deviation (SD) was adopted to express the experimental data.

Supplementary Materials: The following supporting information can be downloaded at: https://www.mdpi.com/article/10.3390/antibiotics13010013/s1. Figure S1: Growth curves of H37Ra (WT) and H37Ra Δ*thyA* (*thyA*$^-$) in liquid culture at 37 °C. The OD_{600} was measured by using a SynergyH1 Hybrid reader (BioTek, USA). Data represent the means of three biological replicates, and error bars denote the standard deviations; Figure S2: Comparison of the transcriptional level of the *ribD* gene during the exponential phase in H37Ra (WT) and H37Ra Δ*thyA* (*thyA*$^-$) by RNA-seq. ns, no significance; Table S1: Collection parameters of multiple reaction monitoring (MRM); Table S2: Mutation analysis of *ribD* in ThyA or DfrA deficient *M. tuberculosis* isolates; Table S3: Plasmids, strains, and primers used in this study.

Author Contributions: J.-F.Y.: Conceptualization, Methodology, Investigation, Writing—Original Draft, Visualization. J.-T.X.: Investigation, Methodology, Visualization. A.F.: Investigation, Validation. B.-L.Q.: Methodology, Visualization. J.G.: Validation, Supervision. X.-E.Z.: Conceptualization, Resources, Writing—Review and Editing, Funding Acquisition. J.-Y.D.: Conceptualization, Resources, Supervision, Writing—Review and Editing, Funding Acquisition. All authors have read and agreed to the published version of the manuscript.

Funding: This work was supported by the National Key Research and Development Program of China (Grant no. 2021YFA1300901 to J.-Y.D.) and the Strategic Priority Research Program of the Chinese Academy of Sciences (Grant no. XDB29020000 to J.-Y.D. and X.-E.Z.).

Institutional Review Board Statement: Not applicable.

Informed Consent Statement: Not applicable.

Data Availability Statement: Data will be made available on request.

Acknowledgments: We thank Chongqing Public Health Medical Center for providing the PAS resistant *M. tuberculosis* clinical isolate with *thyA* R235P mutation.

Conflicts of Interest: The authors declare no conflict of interest.

References

1. World Health Organization (WHO). *Global Tuberculosis Report 2022*; World Health Organization: Geneva, Switzerland, 2022.
2. Thibault, P. Rifampicine, new antitubercular drug. *Presse Med.* **1967**, *75*, 2816.
3. Hosseiniporgham, S.; Sechi, L.A. A Review on Mycobacteriophages: From Classification to Applications. *Pathogens* **2022**, *11*, 777. [CrossRef] [PubMed]
4. Bermingham, A.; Derrick, J.P. The folic acid biosynthesis pathway in bacteria: Evaluation of potential for antibacterial drug discovery. *Bioessays* **2002**, *24*, 637–648. [CrossRef] [PubMed]
5. Chakraborty, S.; Gruber, T.; Barry, C.E., 3rd; Boshoff, H.I.; Rhee, K.Y. *Para*-aminosalicylic acid acts as an alternative substrate of folate metabolism in *Mycobacterium tuberculosis*. *Science* **2013**, *339*, 88–91. [CrossRef] [PubMed]
6. Lehmann, J. *Para*-aminosalicylic acid in the treatment of tuberculosis. *Lancet* **1946**, *1*, 15. [CrossRef] [PubMed]
7. Zumla, A.; Nahid, P.; Cole, S.T. Advances in the development of new tuberculosis drugs and treatment regimens. *Nat. Rev. Drug Discov.* **2013**, *12*, 388–404. [CrossRef] [PubMed]
8. Zheng, J.; Rubin, E.J.; Bifani, P.; Mathys, V.; Lim, V.; Au, M.; Jang, J.; Nam, J.; Dick, T.; Walker, J.R.; et al. *para*-Aminosalicylic acid is a prodrug targeting dihydrofolate reductase in *Mycobacterium tuberculosis*. *J. Biol. Chem.* **2013**, *288*, 23447–23456. [CrossRef]
9. Zhang, X.; Liu, L.; Zhang, Y.; Dai, G.; Huang, H.; Jin, Q. Genetic determinants involved in p-aminosalicylic acid resistance in clinical isolates from tuberculosis patients in northern China from 2006 to 2012. *Antimicrob. Agents Chemother.* **2015**, *59*, 1320–1324. [CrossRef]
10. Zhao, F.; Wang, X.D.; Erber, L.N.; Luo, M.; Guo, A.Z.; Yang, S.S.; Gu, J.; Turman, B.J.; Gao, Y.R.; Li, D.F.; et al. Binding pocket alterations in dihydrofolate synthase confer resistance to *para*-aminosalicylic acid in clinical isolates of *Mycobacterium tuberculosis*. *Antimicrob. Agents Chemother.* **2014**, *58*, 1479–1487. [CrossRef]
11. Yu, J.F.; Xu, J.T.; Yang, S.S.; Gao, M.N.; Si, H.R.; Xiong, D.Y.; Gu, J.; Wu, Z.L.; Zhou, J.; Deng, J.Y. Decreased Methylenetetrahydrofolate Reductase Activity Leads to Increased Sensitivity to *para*-Aminosalicylic Acid in *Mycobacterium tuberculosis*. *Antimicrob. Agents Chemother.* **2022**, *66*, e0146521. [CrossRef]
12. Mathys, V.; Wintjens, R.; Lefevre, P.; Bertout, J.; Singhal, A.; Kiass, M.; Kurepina, N.; Wang, X.M.; Mathema, B.; Baulard, A.; et al. Molecular genetics of *para*-aminosalicylic acid resistance in clinical isolates and spontaneous mutants of *Mycobacterium tuberculosis*. *Antimicrob. Agents Chemother.* **2009**, *53*, 2100–2109. [CrossRef] [PubMed]
13. Rengarajan, J.; Sassetti, C.M.; Naroditskaya, V.; Sloutsky, A.; Bloom, B.R.; Rubin, E.J. The folate pathway is a target for resistance to the drug *para*-aminosalicylic acid (PAS) in mycobacteria. *Mol. Microbiol.* **2004**, *53*, 275–282. [CrossRef] [PubMed]
14. Luo, M.; Li, K.; Zhang, H.; Yan, X.; Gu, J.; Zhang, Z.; Chen, Y.; Li, J.; Wang, J.; Chen, Y. Molecular characterization of *para*-aminosalicylic acid resistant *Mycobacterium tuberculosis* clinical isolates in southwestern China. *Infect. Drug Resist.* **2019**, *12*, 2269–2275. [CrossRef] [PubMed]
15. Fivian-Hughes, A.S.; Houghton, J.; Davis, E.O. *Mycobacterium tuberculosis* thymidylate synthase gene *thyX* is essential and potentially bifunctional, while *thyA* deletion confers resistance to p-aminosalicylic acid. *Microbiology* **2012**, *158*, 308–318. [CrossRef]
16. Carreras, C.W.; Santi, D.V. The catalytic mechanism and structure of thymidylate synthase. *Annu. Rev. Biochem.* **1995**, *64*, 721–762. [CrossRef]
17. Kuhn, P.; Lesley, S.A.; Mathews, I.I.; Canaves, J.M.; Brinen, L.S.; Dai, X.; Deacon, A.M.; Elsliger, M.A.; Eshaghi, S.; Floyd, R.; et al. Crystal structure of thy1, a thymidylate synthase complementing protein from *Thermotoga maritima* at 2.25 A resolution. *Proteins* **2002**, *49*, 142–145. [CrossRef]
18. Bognar, A.L.; Osborne, C.; Shane, B.; Singer, S.C.; Ferone, R. Folylpoly-gamma-glutamate synthetase-dihydrofolate synthetase. Cloning and high expression of the *Escherichia coli* folC gene and purification and properties of the gene product. *J. Biol. Chem.* **1985**, *260*, 5625–5630. [CrossRef]
19. Bognar, A.L.; Shane, B. Bacterial folylpoly(gamma-glutamate) synthase-dihydrofolate synthase. *Methods Enzymol.* **1986**, *122*, 349–359. [CrossRef]
20. Brown, G.M.; Williamson, J.M. Biosynthesis of riboflavin, folic acid, thiamine, and pantothenic acid. *Adv. Enzymol. Relat. Areas Mol. Biol.* **1982**, *53*, 345–381. [CrossRef]
21. Green, J.M.; Matthews, R.G. Folate Biosynthesis, Reduction, and Polyglutamylation and the Interconversion of Folate Derivatives. *EcoSal Plus* **2007**, *2*. [CrossRef]
22. Moradigaravand, D.; Grandjean, L.; Martinez, E.; Li, H.; Zheng, J.; Coronel, J.; Moore, D.; Török, M.E.; Sintchenko, V.; Huang, H.; et al. *dfrA thyA* Double Deletion in *para*-Aminosalicylic Acid-Resistant *Mycobacterium tuberculosis* Beijing Strains. *Antimicrob. Agents Chemother.* **2016**, *60*, 3864–3867. [CrossRef] [PubMed]
23. Cheng, Y.S.; Sacchettini, J.C. Structural Insights into *Mycobacterium tuberculosis* Rv2671 Protein as a Dihydrofolate Reductase Functional Analogue Contributing to *para*-Aminosalicylic Acid Resistance. *Biochemistry* **2016**, *55*, 1107–1119. [CrossRef] [PubMed]
24. Zhang, H.; Li, D.; Zhao, L.; Fleming, J.; Lin, N.; Wang, T.; Liu, Z.; Li, C.; Galwey, N.; Deng, J.; et al. Genome sequencing of 161 *Mycobacterium tuberculosis* isolates from China identifies genes and intergenic regions associated with drug resistance. *Nat. Genet.* **2013**, *45*, 1255–1260. [CrossRef] [PubMed]
25. Hajian, B.; Scocchera, E.; Shoen, C.; Krucinska, J.; Viswanathan, K.; G-Dayanandan, N.; Erlandsen, H.; Estrada, A.; Mikušová, K.; Korduláková, J.; et al. Drugging the Folate Pathway in *Mycobacterium tuberculosis*: The Role of Multi-targeting Agents. *Cell Chem. Biol.* **2019**, *26*, 781–791.e786. [CrossRef]

26. Bardarov, S.; Bardarov, S.; Pavelka, M.S.; Sambandamurthy, V.; Larsen, M.; Tufariello, J.; Chan, J.; Hatfull, G.; Jacobs, W.R. Specialized transduction: An efficient method for generating marked and unmarked targeted gene disruptions in *Mycobacterium tuberculosis*, *M. bovis* BCG and *M. smegmatis*. *Microbiology* **2002**, *148*, 3007–3017. [CrossRef]
27. Martinez, E.; Holmes, N.; Jelfs, P.; Sintchenko, V. Genome sequencing reveals novel deletions associated with secondary resistance to pyrazinamide in MDR *Mycobacterium tuberculosis*. *J. Antimicrob. Chemother.* **2015**, *70*, 2511–2514. [CrossRef]

antibiotics

MDPI

Article

Neonatal Bloodstream Infection with Ceftazidime-Avibactam-Resistant *bla*$_{KPC-2}$-Producing *Klebsiella pneumoniae* Carrying *bla*$_{VEB-25}$

Charalampos Zarras [1,2], Elias Iosifidis [3,4,*], Maria Simitsopoulou [3,4], Styliani Pappa [2], Angeliki Kontou [5], Emmanuel Roilides [3,4] and Anna Papa [2]

1 Microbiology Department, Hippokration Hospital, 54642 Thessaloniki, Greece; zarraschak6@gmail.com
2 Department of Microbiology, School of Medicine, Faculty of Health Sciences, Aristotle University of Thessaloniki, 54124 Thessaloniki, Greece; s_pappa@hotmail.com (S.P.); annap@auth.gr (A.P.)
3 Infectious Disease Unit, 3rd Department of Pediatrics, School of Medicine, Faculty of Health Sciences, Hippokration Hospital, 54642 Thessaloniki, Greece; simitsop@auth.gr (M.S.); roilides@auth.gr (E.R.)
4 Basic and Translational Research Unit, Special Unit for Biomedical Research and Education, School of Medicine, Faculty of Health Sciences, Aristotle University of Thessaloniki, 54124 Thessaloniki, Greece
5 1st Department of Neonatology, School of Medicine, Faculty of Health Sciences, Aristotle University of Thessaloniki, 54124 Thessaloniki, Greece; angiekon2001@yahoo.gr
* Correspondence: iosifidish@auth.gr

Abstract: Background: Although ceftazidime/avibactam (CAZ/AVI) has become an important option for treating adults and children, no data or recommendations exist for neonates. We report a neonatal sepsis case due to CAZ/AVI-resistant *bla*$_{KPC-2}$-harboring *Klebsiella pneumoniae* carrying *bla*$_{VEB-25}$ and the use of a customized active surveillance program in conjunction with enhanced infection control measures. Methods: The index case was an extremely premature neonate hospitalized for 110 days that had been previously treated with multiple antibiotics. Customized molecular surveillance was implemented at hospital level and enhanced infection control measures were taken for early recognition and prevention of outbreak. Detection and identification of *bla*$_{VEB-25}$ was performed using next-generation sequencing. Results: This was the first case of a bloodstream infection caused by KPC-producing *K. pneumoniae* that was resistant to CAZ/AVI without the presence of a metalo-β-lactamase in the multiplex PCR platform in a neonate. All 36 additional patients tested (12 in the same NICU and 24 from other hospital departments) carried wild-type *bla*$_{VEB-1}$ but they did not harbor *bla*$_{VEB-25}$. Conclusion: The emergence of *bla*$_{VEB-25}$ is signal for the horizontal transfer of plasmids at hospital facilities and it is of greatest concern for maintaining a sharp vigilance for the surveillance of novel resistance mechanisms. Molecular diagnostics can guide appropriate antimicrobial therapy and the early implementation of infection control measures against antimicrobial resistance.

Keywords: multidrug resistance; Gram-negative bacteria; *Enterobacterales*; carbapenemases; *bla*$_{VEB-25}$ carbapenemase; neonatal intensive care unit

1. Introduction

Antimicrobial resistance (AMR) is a public health threat facing humanity as it tests the resilience of health systems worldwide [1,2]. Various genetic elements are associated with the development of resistance because they manage via complex pathways to be transmitted between bacteria [3]. In addition, other practices such as delayed and/or incorrect diagnosis and the prescription of broad-spectrum antibiotics reinforce the problem of AMR [4]. Advances and innovations in the whole genome sequencing method and the bioinformatics revolution contribute to the immediate detection of the causes of resistance and the taking of timely and effective control measures [5].

A decisive factor in the development of AMR in healthcare facilities and especially in the intensive care units (ICU) of hospitals is the spread of multiresistant Gram-negative bacteria. *Enterobacterales* are the most important, among which *Klebsiella pneumoniae* is the main representative. *K. pneumoniae* is the second most common Gram-negative opportunistic pathogen and one of the most prevalent causes of community- and hospital-acquired infections [6]. It is responsible for health-care-associated pneumonia [7] and bacterial neonatal sepsis in low- and middle-income countries [8]. A serious public health threat is the emergence and dissemination of carbapenem-resistant *K. pneumoniae* (CRKP) that is associated with high morbidity and mortality, increased medical costs, and prolonged hospital stay [9]. In addition, CRKP infections affect disability-adjusted life years (DALYs) per 100,000 population with a median value in the European Union of 11.5 years, while for these infections treatment options are limited [10,11]. CRKP isolates have a variety of mechanisms, which may confer resistance to virtually all available β-lactam antibacterial drugs, including carbapenems. The main resistance molecular mechanism is the production of a range of carbapenemases, including KPC, NDM, VIM, and OXA-48-like carbapenemases [12,13]. KPC-producing CRKP strains display the most extensive global distribution and represent a significant challenge due to their limited therapeutic options [14].

A novel β-lactam/β-lactamase inhibitor (BL/BLIs) combination is effective against strains of non-metallo-β lactamase producing *Enterobacterales* (Ambler class A, class C, and some class D β-lactamases) [15,16]. Ceftazidime/avibactam (CAZ/AVI) [17] has become an important first-line option for treating adult and pediatric (>3 months of age) patients with serious infections caused by carbapenem-resistant organisms, but not yet for neonates (IDSA) [18]. It is indicated for the treatment of complicated intra-abdominal and urinary tract infections, and infections caused by carbapenem-resistant *Enterobacterales* (CRE) or carbapenem-resistant *Pseudomonas aeruginosa*, in patients with limited or no other treatment options [19].

Although KPC-producing *Enterobacterales* strains are generally considered susceptible to CAZ/AVI, isolates resistant to this antimicrobial agent have been documented without the evidence of metallo-β-lactamases [20]. In 2018, a rapid risk assessment conducted by ECDC identified CAZ/AVI resistance in CRE as a public health threat that merits careful monitoring [21]. CAZ/AVI resistance mechanisms include the increased expression of the bla_{KPC} gene product (acquisition of resistance was mostly associated with isolates harboring the substitution D179Y in $bla_{\mathrm{KPC\text{-}3}}$ or in $bla_{\mathrm{KPC\text{-}2}}$) [22,23], the presence of other genetic determinants of resistance against ESBL-producing *Enterobacterales* (SHV-, CTX-M-, or VEB-type β-lactamases) [24,25], changes in cell permeability (i.e., non-functional porins-OmpK35, OmpK36, and OmpK37) [26], and the expression of efflux pumps [27].

VEB-type β-lactamases (Vietnamese extended-spectrum β-lactamase) are a group of Ambler class A enzymes inhibited by avibactam. $bla_{\mathrm{VEB\text{-}25}}$ differs from $bla_{\mathrm{VEB\text{-}1}}$ by a missense mutation (substitution of lysine with arginine at position 237 -K234R) [28], which compromises the inhibitory efficiency of avibactam [29].

Herein, we report a successful treatment of bloodstream infection associated with CAZ/AVI-resistant $bla_{\mathrm{KPC\text{-}2}}$-producing *K. pneumoniae* carrying $bla_{\mathrm{VEB\text{-}25}}$ in a preterm neonate hospitalized in the neonatal intensive care unit (NICU) of a tertiary hospital and the use of a customized active surveillance program in conjunction with infection control measures for the early recognition and prevention of an outbreak.

2. Results

2.1. Index Case

The index case was the first neonate of a twin pregnancy born to a 33-year-old healthy primigravida at gestational age of $25w^{+5d}$ (birth weight = 850 gr, appropriate for a gestational age neonate) due to the premature rapture of membranes and the onset of labor. Postnatally, the patient presented respiratory distress syndrome, patent ductus arteriosus, severe bronchopulmonary dysplasia and need for prolonged mechanical ventilation, posthemorrhagic ventricular dilation, gastro-oesophageal reflux disease, retinopathy of prematurity, and episodes of late onset sepsis (LOS). The first LOS occurred on the fourth day of life due to carbapenem-resistant *Acinetobacter baumannii*, which was successfully treated. The patient was colonized with carbapenem-resistant *A. baumannii* and *Providencia stuartii* between Day 4 and 25, respectively. During that time, the neonate had been exposed to multiple antibiotic regimens for prolonged time periods, including meropenem, aminoglycosides, colistin, tigecycline, and CAZ/AVI due to episodes of suspected LOS and colonization by CR Gram-negative bacteria.

At Day 108, the neonate was on nasal continuous positive airway pressure due to chronic lung disease, and presented with fever and impaired peripheral perfusion. Empiric antibiotic treatment with colistin (300,000 IU/kg/day every 8 h), tigecycline (2 mg/kg/day every 12 h) and daptomycin (10 mg/kg/day once daily) was immediately initiated for suspected sepsis and due to the previous administration of multiple antimicrobial regimens. Blood culture was positive for a Gram-negative rod within 24 h since the onset of symptoms. A multiplex PCR platform (Biofire® FilmArray®, Biomeriuex, Marcy-l'Étoile, France) was used within an hour from positive blood culture. A bla_{KPC} producing *K. pneumoniae* was detected and CAZ/AVI at a reduced dose of 31 mg/kg/d every 8 h was added to the antimicrobial regimen in attendance of the Antimicrobial Susceptibility Testing (AST).

During the first 48 h of this sepsis episode, the neonate deteriorated, requiring mechanical ventilation and possessing high inflammatory indices (max CRP value of 394 mg/L) and thrombocytopenia. At Day 110, the AST displayed a high level of resistance to almost all antimicrobial agents, including piperacillin/tazobactam, cefepime, cefoxitin, ceftazidime, ceftriaxone, imipenem, meropenem (MIC $\geq$ 16 mg/L), amikacin, gentamicin, ampicillin/sulbactam, aztreonam, ciprofloxacin, levofloxacin, fosfomycin, and trimethoprim/sulfamethoxazole. It was also resistant to novel agents, like ceftolozane/tazobactam and CAZ/AVI, while it was only susceptible to tigecycline and colistin. The isolate displayed a positive phenyl boronic acid phenotypic test and the lateral flow immunoassay, and the PCR method confirmed that the isolate carried bla_{KPC}.

A favorable clinical and microbiological response was documented including defervescence and a decrease in CRP within 48–72 h, the first negative blood culture within 4 days, and the discontinuation of invasive mechanical ventilation within 8 days of colistin and tigecycline initiation. The administration of both daptomycin and CAZ/AVI was discontinued, whereas ciprofloxacin was empirically added four days after the first positive blood culture for a total of 13 days. The neonate was successfully treated with colistin and tigecycline for a total of 18 days.

NGS Report

A variety of genes conferring resistance to antimicrobial agents and heavy metals, as well as genes related to virulence, capsule, and efflux, and regulator systems were detected (Table 1). Only one serine-carbapenemase was detected, which was the $bla_{KPC\text{-}2}$ gene and belonged to ST35. Another five β-lactamases ($bla_{SHV\text{-}33}$, $bla_{TEM\text{-}1B}$, $bla_{VEB\text{-}25}$, $bla_{DHA\text{-}1}$, and $bla_{OXA\text{-}10}$) were co-detected, including the $bla_{VEB\text{-}25}$. The co-production of $bla_{KPC\text{-}2}$ and $bla_{VEB\text{-}25}$ in *K. pneumoniae* has been associated with CAZ/AVI resistance in the absence of metallo-β-lactamase [24].

Table 1. Genetic characteristics of the neonatal blood *K. pneumoniae* isolate of the study via NGS.

Strain ID	A1746/22
Date of isolation	25 February 2022
Biological sample	Blood
MLST	35
Plasmids	IncC, IncR, IncFIA(HI1), IncFIB(K), IncFIB(pKPHS1), IncFIB(pQil), IncFII(K)

Table 1. *Cont.*

Strain ID		A1746/22
Antibiotic Resistance	β-lactamases	SHV-33, TEM-1B, VEB-25, DHA-1, OXA-10
	Carbapenemases	KPC-2
	Aminoglycosides	ant(2″)-Ia, aph(3″)-Ib, aph(6)-Id, rmtB, aadA1
	Quinolone	qnrB4, oqxA, oqxB
	Fosfomycin	fosA
	Sulfonamide	sul1, sul2
	Phenicol	catA1, cmlA1
	Tetracycline	tet(A), tet(G)
Resistance to Heavy Metals		merC, merP, merT, silR
Virulence		kfuA, mrkA, mrkF, mrkH, mrkl, ybtE, ybtQ, ybtT, ybtX
Capsule		wzi
Efflux and Regulator Systems		acrR, envR, fis, marA, marR, oqxR, rob, sdiA, soxR, soxS, ramA, ramR, rarA

2.2. *Molecular and Phenotypic Surveillance within the NICU and the Hospital*

Thirteen *K. pneumoniae* strains were isolated from stool samples of neonates hospitalized in the NICU within a period of 3 months upon the recognition of the index case. Among these isolates, only the index case was *bla*$_{VEB-25}$ positive (Figure 1A), confirming the NGS result. Based on the AST results, 24 additional carbapenem-resistant *K. pneumoniae* strains collected from various hospital sites were also analyzed with targeted PCR; even though they contained *bla*$_{VEB-1}$, they did not harbor *bla*$_{VEB-25}$ (Figure 1B).

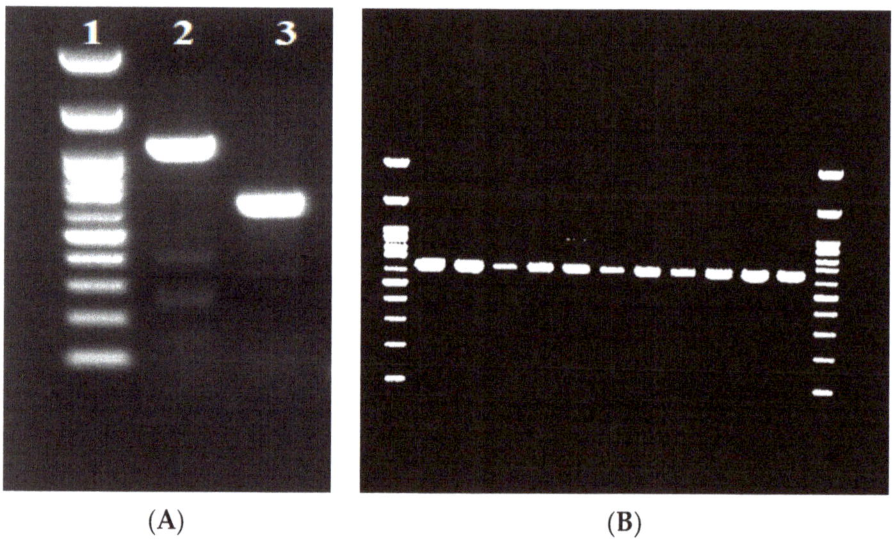

Figure 1. Agarose gel electrophoresis profile of the *bla*$_{VEB-25}$ variant. Panel (**A**) shows the *bla*$_{VEB-25}$ positive variant, whereas panel (**B**) shows the 642 bp amplified products of *bla*$_{VEB-25}$-negative carbapenem-resistant *K. pneumoniae* strains. The amplified products of 1070 bp and 642 bp were produced using the external VEBcas-F/VEBcas-B (lane 2) and internal VEB-F/VEB-B primer pairs (lane 3). The amplified product containing the entire gene (1070 bp) was used to deduce the nucleotide sequence. The 100 bp DNA ladder with reference bands ranging from 100 bp to 1500 bp is indicated in lane 1.

Based on the AST results of the 24 carbapenem-resistant *K. pneumoniae* strains collected from various hospital sites, half were characterized as pan-drug-resistant [PDR, non-susceptibility to all agents in all antimicrobial categories (i.e., bacterial isolates are not susceptible to any clinically available drug)], and the other half as extensively drug resistant [XDR, non-susceptibility to at least one agent in all but two or fewer antimicrobial categories (i.e., bacterial isolates remain susceptible to only one or two antimicrobial categories)]. Therefore, all 24 CRKP isolates displayed high levels of resistance to almost all antimicrobials including imipenem (MIC $\geq$ 16 mg/L), meropenem (MIC $\geq$ 16 mg/L), amikacin (MIC $\geq$ 16 mg/L), gentamicin (MIC $\geq$ 16 mg/L), ampicillin/sulbactam (MIC $\geq$ 32 mg/L), piperacillin/tazobactam (MIC $\geq$ 128 mg/L), aztreonam (MIC $\geq$ 64 mg/L), cefepime (MIC $\geq$ 64 mg/L), cefoxitin (MIC $\geq$ 64 mg/L), ceftazidime (MIC $\geq$ 64 mg/L), ceftriaxone (MIC $\geq$ 64 mg/L), ciprofloxacin (MIC $\geq$ 4 mg/L), levofloxacin (MIC $\geq$ 8 mg/L), fosfomycin (MIC $\geq$ 256 mg/L), and trimethoprim/sulfamethoxazole (MIC $\geq$ 320 mg/L). These isolates were also analyzed with targeted PCR; even though they contained $bla_{\text{VEB-1}}$, they did not harbor $bla_{\text{VEB-25}}$.

2.3. Overall Assessment

This index case was the last neonate that was infected with *A. baumannii* and colonized by *P. stuartii* within the NICU after the implementation of enhanced infection control measures targeting these two pathogens. Upon the recognition of the first *K. pneumoniae* producing $bla_{\text{KPC-2}}$ and $bla_{\text{VEB-25}}$ and a combination of intensified and targeted infection control actions in the unit, there were no other cases within the NICU for the next 6 months.

3. Discussion

We report a neonatal case of a bloodstream infection caused by a *K. pneumoniae* strain co-producing $bla_{\text{KPC-2}}$ and $bla_{\text{VEB-25}}$ β-lactamases and emphasize the use of precise medicine to customize infection control measures. Treatment options for infections caused by carbapenem-resistant bacteria are extremely limited in neonates. The "off label" use of either "last-line" antimicrobial agents (such as polymyxins and tigecycline) or the currently available newer β-lactam/β-lactam inhibitor combinations, such as CAZ/AVI, meropenem-vaborbactam, and imipenem cilastatin-relebactam that are not yet licensed for neonates, for the empirical treatment of neonatal sepsis in areas endemic for CRKP is still questionable due to limited pharmacokinetic data and local epidemiology of resistant genes [30].

One of the mechanisms that confers resistance to CAZ/AVI is the new bla_{KPC} variants that are constantly appearing worldwide. Very recently, Shi et al. reported multiple novel variants in a *K. pneumoniae* strain carrying $bla_{\text{KPC-2}}$ from two separate patients during their exposure to CAZ/AVI. In one patient, the $bla_{\text{KPC-2}}$ mutated to $bla_{\text{KPC-35}}$, $bla_{\text{KPC-78}}$, and $bla_{\text{KPC-33}}$ during the same period, while in the other patient it mutated to $bla_{\text{KPC-79}}$ and $bla_{\text{KPC-76}}$, thus enhancing the level of resistance [31]. ST258 *K. pneumoniae* is considered the most frequent type in the majority of bla_{KPC}-associated infections resistant to CAZ/AVI [32].

The $bla_{\text{KPC-2}}$-harboring *K. pneumoniae* isolated in our study belonged to Sequence Type ST35. To the best of our knowledge, this is the first report of ST35 CRKP bearing both $bla_{\text{KPC-2}}$ and $bla_{\text{VEB-25}}$ that confers resistance to CAZ/AVI. Findlay et al. identified two isolates as belonging to Sequence Types ST147 and ST258, harboring $bla_{\text{VEB-25}}$ on the plasmid, that confer resistance to CAZ/AVI [33].

To date, there are three reports of CAZ/AVI-resistant KPC-producing *K. pneumoniae* emergence in Greece, all in adults (six infected and five colonized patients) [24,34,35]. Notably, the first CAZ/AVI-resistant clinical isolate was detected in Greece before the introduction of CAZ/AVI in clinical practice. The resistance was due to the existence of $bla_{\text{KPC-23}}$ (variant differed from $bla_{\text{KPC-3}}$ by one -V240A, and from $bla_{\text{KPC-2}}$ by two amino acid substitutions -V240A and H274Y) [34]. CAZ/AVI resistance due to the harboring of $bla_{\text{VEB-25}}$ has been reported in two additional cases (one isolate from blood and one from the lower respiratory tract) from patients without prior CAZ/AVI exposure [35]. Eight more CAZ/AVI-resistant CRKP isolates were detected in patients not previously exposed to

CAZ/AVI (two patients with catheter-related bloodstream infections, one with ventilator-associated pneumonia, and five with colonization); the resistance was conferred by the harboring $bla_{\text{VEB-25}}$ and $bla_{\text{VEB-14}}$ [24]. After intense epidemiological and microbiological surveillance in our NICU, as well as in pediatric and adult departments within our general hospital (especially pediatric and adult intensive care units), we could not find the source of this resistant organism. However, our index patient had been previously exposed to multiple courses of antimicrobial agents, including CAZ/AVI, and also had gut colonization with XDR Gram-negative bacteria, such as *A. baumannii* and *P. stuartii*.

This was the first premature neonate presenting with sepsis due to CAZ/AVI-resistant $bla_{\text{KPC-2}}$-harboring *K. pneumoniae* carrying the $bla_{\text{VEB-25}}$ that was successfully treated with non-conventional "off-label" antimicrobial agents. Currently, available diagnostic platforms detect the presence of the most prevalent carbapenemases, such as KPC, VIM, NDM, and OXA. Neonatologists and infectious disease specialists should be cautious when interpreting the results from these molecular platforms for decision making in empiric and targeted treatment for neonatal sepsis. The mechanism of resistance, especially for the newer β-lactam/β-lactamase inhibitors, may differ in times and in different parts of the world and even within the same institution [36]. In addition, various mechanisms of CAZ/AVI resistance emphasize the need for the surveillance of CAZ/AVI-resistant pathogens, as well as for its judicious use.

4. Materials and Methods

4.1. Risk Assessment and Bundle of Actions Taken after Index Case

This was the first case of a bloodstream infection caused by KPC-producing *K. pneumoniae* that was resistant to CAZ/AVI without the presence of metalo-β-lactamase in the multiplex PCR platform in a neonate. The bundle of actions implemented is summarized in Figure 2 and included: (1) enhanced infection control measures including strict isolation of the case index; (2) continuation of active surveillance for CRE and tests for CAZ/AVI susceptibility reported for all isolates recovered from surveillance; (3) application of next-generation sequencing (NGS) and molecular testing for the index case to identify probable mechanism(s) of CAZ/AVI resistance; (4) targeted PCR analysis in all CRE isolates from all neonates in the ICU, independently to CAZ/AVI susceptibility; and (5) targeted PCR analysis specifically for CAZ/AVI-R isolates from other departments of the hospital to identify potential sources and/or burden of a potential outbreak.

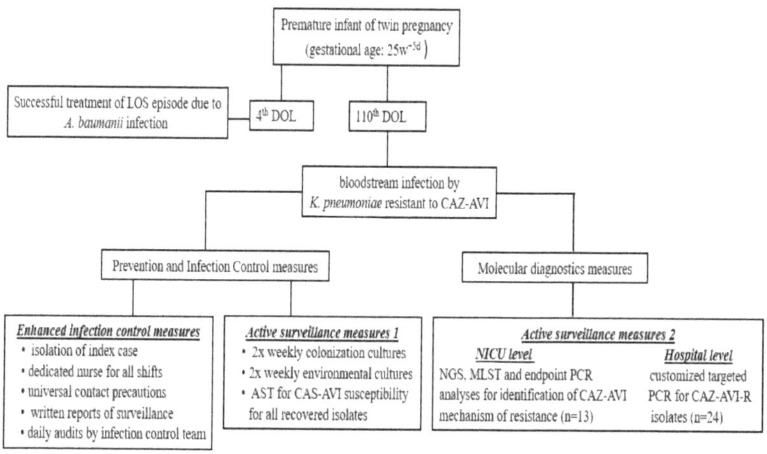

Figure 2. Summary of a bundle of actions followed in a premature neonate with a ceftazidime-avibactam-resistant KPC-2-producing *Klebsiella pneumoniae* bloodstream infection carrying the VEB-25 gene. LOS: late onset sepsis, DOL: day of life, CAZ-AVI: ceftazidime-avibactam.

4.1.1. Infection Control Measures

The NICU was already on strict infection control measures, including the cohorting of all neonates colonized/infected with an XDR *A. baumannii* strain. Upon recognition of this index case, extra measures were taken: isolation of index case, dedicated nurse for all shifts, universal application of contact precautions, written reports of active surveillance, and daily audits by infection control team (with a dedicated infection control nurse and a dedicated pediatric infectious disease specialist).

4.1.2. Active Surveillance

Already in place with twice weekly colonization cultures. Specifically, stool samples were taken from the neonates on the NICU and cultured on MacConkey agar plates supplemented with 1 mg/L meropenem. AST was applied to all isolates as written in Section 4.2, including CAZ/AVI susceptibility. Active surveillance included not only gut and pharyngeal colonization but also environmental cultures.

4.2. Microbiological Methods, Antimicrobial Susceptibility Testing, and Phenotypic Analysis

CRKP was identified with a VITEK 2 automated system (Biomeriuex, Marcy-l'Étoile, France) using the GN ID according to the manufacturer's instructions. The AST of *K. pneumoniae* was performed using the AST 376 and XN10 cards; the interpretation of results was according to the European Committee on Antimicrobial Susceptibility Testing (EUCAST) breakpoints of January 2022. Susceptibility testing to CAZ/AVI was performed using MIC test strips (Liofilchem srl, Roseto, Italy), while susceptibility testing to colistin was performed using the broth microdilution method (Liofilchem srl, Roseto degli Abruzzi, Italy). Tigecycline was evaluated using the susceptibility breakpoints approved by the US Food and Drug Administration (MIC $\leq$ 2 mg/L for susceptibility and $\geq$8 mg/L for resistance).

The isolate was phenotypically tested for KPC and metallo-β-lactamase (MBL) production using phenylboronic acid and ethylenediaminetetraacetic acid. Carbapenemase genes bla_{KPC}, bla_{NDM}, $bla_{OXA\text{-}48\text{-}like}$, bla_{IMP}, and bla_{VIM} were screened with a multiplex lateral flow immunoassay (NG-Test CARBA 5, NG Biotech, Guipry, France). The detection limits using purified recombinant enzymes for NDM, KPC, IMP, VIM, and OXA-48-like were 150, 600, 200, 300, and 300 pg/mL, respectively.

4.3. Next-Generation Sequencing (NGS)

DNA was extracted using the DNA extraction kit (Qiagen, Hilden, Germany). The Qubit double-strand DNA HS assay kit (Q32851, Life Technologies Corporation, Grand Island, NY, USA) was used for measuring the dsDNA concentration. All procedures regarding shearing, purification, ligation, barcoding, size selection, library amplification and quantitation, emulsion PCR, and enrichment were conducted according to the manufacturer's guidelines. After template enrichment, sequencing was performed on an Ion PGM™ semiconductor sequencer using a Hi-Q View Sequencing Kit and a 316 Chip V2 BC (Thermo Fisher Scientific, Waltham, MA, USA). The sequence reads were de novo assembled and annotated using Geneious Prime version 2021.2.1. The sequence of the *K. pneumoniae* NTUH-K2044 strain (Accession number NC-012731) was used as reference.

4.4. MLST and Detection of Antimicrobial Resistance Genes and Plasmids

MLST and antimicrobial resistance genes and plasmids were identified using the online databases at the Center for Genomic Epidemiology (MLST-2.0, Resfinder 4.1 and Plasmid finder) [37–44] and the Comprehensive Antibiotic Resistance Database (CARD) Bait Capture Platform 1.0.0 [https://card.mcmaster.ca/ (accessed on 4 August 2023)]. Genes related to virulence, resistance to heavy metals, efflux, regulator systems, and capsules were detected using the Institut Pasteur website on *K. pneumoniae* [https://bigsdb.pasteur.fr/klebsiella/ (accessed on 4 August 2023)].

4.5. Targeted PCR Analysis

Molecular surveillance at the NICU and hospital level: After the recognition of the existence of $bla_{\text{VEB-25}}$ as the mechanism of CAZ/AVI resistance in KPC *K. pneumoniae*, targeted PCR protocol was initiated to investigate transmission within the NICU, but also to other carbapenem-resistant *K. pneumoniae* isolated from other pediatric and adult departments in the hospital (particularly, pediatric and adult intensive care units). A total of 37 *K. pneumoniae* strains were tested for the presence of $bla_{\text{VEB-1}}$. Thirteen of them were isolated from stool samples collected from neonates in the NICU where the $bla_{\text{VEB-25}}$ index case was identified, and twenty-four strains were isolated from different clinical sources (blood, urine, tracheal aspirate, trauma, and central venous catheter) collected from several departments of the hospital to investigate potential sites of outbreak. Plasmid DNA was extracted using the alkaline lysis method, as described previously (H.C.Birnboim and J.Doly NAR 7: 1513-1523, 1979). For PCR amplification, VEB-F (5′-CGA CTT CCA TTT CCC GAT GC-3′) and VEB-B (5′-GGA CTC TGC AAC AAA TAC GC-3′) primers were used as diagnostic primers to amplify a 642 bp internal VEB-1 DNA segment, whereas the external primers VEBcas-F (5′-GTT AGC GGT AAT TTA ACC AGA TAG-3′) and VEBcas-B (5′-CGG TTT GGG CTA TGG GCA G-3′) were used to amplify the entire gene for DNA sequencing. For each PCR reaction, 50–70 ng of *K. pneumoniae* plasmid DNA was used in a standard PCR reaction using Kapa Hi Fi DNA polymerase (KAPA Biosystems) with the following amplification program: 1 cycle of 95 °C 3 min, 35 cycles of 20 s at 94 °C, 30 s at 55 °C, 30 s at 72 °C, and a final extension step of 1 min at 72 °C. The PCR products were Sanger sequenced. Nucleotide sequence analysis and pairwise alignments were performed using the National Center of Biotechnology Information website [https://www.ncbi.nlm.nih.gov accessed on 4 August 2023)].

5. Conclusions

Applying next-generation sequencing technology is crucial for guiding the prediction of underlying resistance mechanisms facilitating the study of the evolution and molecular epidemiology of multidrug-resistant pathogens, especially in endemic areas. The emergence of $bla_{\text{VEB-25}}$ is a warning for the horizontal transfer of plasmids at hospital facilities, and it is of greatest concern for maintaining a sharp vigilance for the surveillance of novel resistance mechanisms. The use of molecular diagnostics may guide appropriate antimicrobial therapy and the early implementation of strict infection control measures, and therefore could play an important role in the fight against antimicrobial resistance.

Author Contributions: C.Z.: investigation, formal analysis, review and editing, and writing the initial draft. E.I.: investigation, formal analysis, review and editing, and writing the initial draft. M.S.: formal analysis and review and editing. S.P.: investigation and review and editing. A.K.: provision of study materials and review and editing. E.R.: methodology, data curation, provision of study materials, formal analysis, review and editing, and supervision. A.P.: conceptualization, methodology, data curation, formal analysis, visualization, review and editing, supervision, and funding acquisition. C.Z., E.I., E.R. and A.P. contributed equally to this work. All authors have read and agreed to the published version of the manuscript.

Funding: This work was supported by the European Union's Horizon 2020 project VEO (grant number 874735).

Institutional Review Board Statement: This study was performed in line with the principles of the Declaration of Helsinki. This study was approved by the Ethics Committee of Aristotle's University Medical Faculty (no. of approval 5.160/18-12-19). Since this was a mainly microbiological retrospective analysis of the bacteria isolated from the index case and during surveillance from other hospitalized patients according to the policy of the Infection Control and Prevention Committee of Hippokration General Hospital, there was no need for informed consent from the parents or the patients.

Informed Consent Statement: Informed consent for publication was signed by the father of the index patient and is available in the medical chart of the patient.

Data Availability Statement: The datasets generated during, and/or analyzed during, the current study are not publicly available due to the fact that these are the results of patient examinations carried out in a public hospital, but are available from the corresponding author on reasonable request.

Acknowledgments: The authors thank the personnel of the NICU that helped obtain surveillance samples from the patients, and the laboratory personnel who helped with the laboratory work. The help of Kostantinos Zarras in the experiments is also greatly acknowledged.

Conflicts of Interest: The authors declare no conflict of interest.

Accession Numbers

The data for this study have been deposited in the European Nucleotide Archive (ENA) at EMBL-EBI under Biosample accession number SAMEA112484914.

References

1. Aljeldah, M.M. Antimicrobial Resistance and Its Spread Is a Global Threat. *Antibiotics* **2022**, *11*, 1082. [CrossRef] [PubMed]
2. Dadgostar, P. Antimicrobial Resistance: Implications and Costs. *Infect. Drug Resist.* **2019**, *12*, 3903–3910. [CrossRef] [PubMed]
3. Reygaert, W.C. An overview of the antimicrobial resistance mechanisms of bacteria. *AIMS Microbiol.* **2018**, *4*, 482–501. [CrossRef] [PubMed]
4. Chaw, P.S.; Hopner, J.; Mikolajczyk, R. The knowledge, attitude and practice of health practitioners towards antibiotic prescribing and resistance in developing countries-A systematic review. *J. Clin. Pharm. Ther.* **2018**, *43*, 606–613. [CrossRef]
5. Schurch, A.C.; van Schaik, W. Challenges and opportunities for whole-genome sequencing-based surveillance of antibiotic resistance. *Ann. N.Y. Acad. Sci.* **2017**, *1388*, 108–120. [CrossRef]
6. Ssekatawa, K.; Byarugaba, D.K.; Nakavuma, J.L.; Kato, C.D.; Ejobi, F.; Tweyongyere, R.; Eddie, W.M. Prevalence of pathogenic Klebsiella pneumoniae based on PCR capsular typing harbouring carbapenemases encoding genes in Uganda tertiary hospitals. *Antimicrob. Resist. Infect. Control.* **2021**, *10*, 57. [CrossRef]
7. Juan, C.H.; Chuang, C.; Chen, C.H.; Li, L.; Lin, Y.T. Clinical characteristics, antimicrobial resistance and capsular types of community-acquired, healthcare-associated, and nosocomial Klebsiella pneumoniae bacteremia. *Antimicrob. Resist. Infect. Control.* **2019**, *8*, 1. [CrossRef]
8. Milton, R.; Gillespie, D.; Dyer, C.; Taiyari, K.; Carvalho, M.J.; Thomson, K.; Sands, K.; Portal, E.A.R.; Hood, K.; Ferreira, A.; et al. Neonatal sepsis and mortality in low-income and middle-income countries from a facility-based birth cohort: An international multisite prospective observational study. *Lancet Glob. Health* **2022**, *10*, e661–e672. [CrossRef]
9. Agyeman, A.A.; Bergen, P.J.; Rao, G.G.; Nation, R.L.; Landersdorfer, C.B. Mortality, clinical and microbiological response following antibiotic therapy among patients with carbapenem-resistant Klebsiella pneumoniae infections (a meta-analysis dataset). *Data Brief* **2020**, *28*, 104907. [CrossRef]
10. Cassini, A.; Plachouras, D.; Monnet, D.L. Attributable deaths caused by infections with antibiotic-resistant bacteria in France–Authors' reply. *Lancet Infect. Dis.* **2019**, *19*, 129–130. [CrossRef]
11. Alexander, B.T.; Marschall, J.; Tibbetts, R.J.; Neuner, E.A.; Dunne, W.M., Jr.; Ritchie, D.J. Treatment and clinical outcomes of urinary tract infections caused by KPC-producing Enterobacteriaceae in a retrospective cohort. *Clin. Ther.* **2012**, *34*, 1314–1323. [CrossRef] [PubMed]
12. Ainoda, Y.; Aoki, K.; Ishii, Y.; Okuda, K.; Furukawa, H.; Manabe, R.; Sahara, T.; Nakamura-Uchiyama, F.; Kurosu, H.; Ando, Y.; et al. Klebsiella pneumoniae carbapenemase (KPC)-producing Klebsiella pneumoniae ST258 isolated from a Japanese patient without a history of foreign travel-a new public health concern in Japan: A case report. *BMC Infect. Dis.* **2019**, *19*, 20. [CrossRef]
13. Mathers, A.J.; Vegesana, K.; German-Mesner, I.; Ainsworth, J.; Pannone, A.; Crook, D.W.; Sifri, C.D.; Sheppard, A.; Stoesser, N.; Peto, T.; et al. Risk factors for Klebsiella pneumoniae carbapenemase (KPC) gene acquisition and clinical outcomes across multiple bacterial species. *J. Hosp. Infect.* **2020**, *104*, 456–468. [CrossRef]
14. Jean, S.S.; Harnod, D.; Hsueh, P.R. Global Threat of Carbapenem-Resistant Gram-Negative Bacteria. *Front. Cell. Infect. Microbiol.* **2022**, *12*, 823684. [CrossRef]
15. Sherry, N.; Howden, B. Emerging Gram negative resistance to last-line antimicrobial agents fosfomycin, colistin and ceftazidime-avibactam-epidemiology, laboratory detection and treatment implications. *Expert Rev. Anti-Infect. Ther.* **2018**, *16*, 289–306. [CrossRef]
16. Coskun, Y.; Atici, S. Successful Treatment of Pandrug-resistant Klebsiella pneumoniae Infection With Ceftazidime-avibactam in a Preterm Infant: A Case Report. *Pediatr. Infect. Dis. J.* **2020**, *39*, 854–856. [CrossRef]
17. U.S. Food and Drug Administration. *FDA Approves New Antibacterial Drug Avycaz*; FDA news release; U.S. FDA: Silver Spring, MD, USA, 2015.
18. Tamma, P.D.; Aitken, S.L.; Bonomo, R.A.; Mathers, A.J.; van Duin, D.; Clancy, C.J. Infectious Diseases Society of America 2022 Guidance on the Treatment of Extended-Spectrum beta-lactamase Producing Enterobacterales (ESBL-E), Carbapenem-Resistant Enterobacterales (CRE), and Pseudomonas aeruginosa with Difficult-to-Treat Resistance (DTR-P. aeruginosa). *Clin. Infect. Dis.* **2022**, *75*, 187–212. [CrossRef]

19. van Duin, D.; Bonomo, R.A. Ceftazidime/Avibactam and Ceftolozane/Tazobactam: Second-generation beta-Lactam/beta-Lactamase Inhibitor Combinations. *Clin. Infect. Dis.* **2016**, *63*, 234–241. [CrossRef]
20. Di Bella, S.; Giacobbe, D.R.; Maraolo, A.E.; Viaggi, V.; Luzzati, R.; Bassetti, M.; Luzzaro, F.; Principe, L. Resistance to ceftazidime/avibactam in infections and colonisations by KPC-producing Enterobacterales: A systematic review of observational clinical studies. *J. Glob. Antimicrob. Resist.* **2021**, *25*, 268–281. [CrossRef]
21. ECDC. *Emergence of Resistance to Ceftazidime-Avibactam in Carbapenem-Resistant Enterobacteriaceae-12 June 2018*; ECDC: Stockholm, Sweden, 2018.
22. Hemarajata, P.; Humphries, R.M. Ceftazidime/avibactam resistance associated with L169P mutation in the omega loop of KPC-2. *J. Antimicrob. Chemother.* **2019**, *74*, 1241–1243. [CrossRef]
23. Haidar, G.; Clancy, C.J.; Shields, R.K.; Hao, B.; Cheng, S.; Nguyen, M.H. Mutations in blaKPC-3 That Confer Ceftazidime-Avibactam Resistance Encode Novel KPC-3 Variants That Function as Extended-Spectrum beta-Lactamases. *Antimicrob. Agents Chemother.* **2017**, *61*, e02245-21. [CrossRef] [PubMed]
24. Galani, I.; Karaiskos, I.; Souli, M.; Papoutsaki, V.; Galani, L.; Gkoufa, A.; Antoniadou, A.; Giamarellou, H. Outbreak of KPC-2-producing Klebsiella pneumoniae endowed with ceftazidime-avibactam resistance mediated through a VEB-1-mutant (VEB-25), Greece, September to October 2019. *Euro Surveill.* **2020**, *25*, 2000028. [CrossRef] [PubMed]
25. Castanheira, M.; Simner, P.J.; Bradford, P.A. Extended-spectrum beta-lactamases: An update on their characteristics, epidemiology and detection. *JAC-Antimicrob. Resist.* **2021**, *3*, dlab092. [CrossRef] [PubMed]
26. Humphries, R.M.; Hemarajata, P. Resistance to Ceftazidime-Avibactam in Klebsiella pneumoniae Due to Porin Mutations and the Increased Expression of KPC-3. *Antimicrob. Agents Chemother.* **2017**, *61*, 10–128. [CrossRef] [PubMed]
27. Nelson, K.; Hemarajata, P.; Sun, D.; Rubio-Aparicio, D.; Tsivkovski, R.; Yang, S.; Sebra, R.; Kasarskis, A.; Nguyen, H.; Hanson, B.M.; et al. Resistance to Ceftazidime-Avibactam Is Due to Transposition of KPC in a Porin-Deficient Strain of Klebsiella pneumoniae with Increased Efflux Activity. *Antimicrob. Agents Chemother.* **2017**, *61*, e00989-17. [CrossRef]
28. Protonotariou, E.; Meletis, G.; Pilalas, D.; Mantzana, P.; Tychala, A.; Kotzamanidis, C.; Papadopoulou, D.; Papadopoulos, T.; Polemis, M.; Metallidis, S.; et al. Polyclonal Endemicity of Carbapenemase-Producing Klebsiella pneumoniae in ICUs of a Greek Tertiary Care Hospital. *Antibiotics* **2022**, *11*, 149. [CrossRef]
29. Lahiri, S.D.; Alm, R.A. Identification of Novel VEB beta-Lactamase Enzymes and Their Impact on Avibactam Inhibition. *Antimicrob. Agents Chemother.* **2016**, *60*, 3183–3186. [CrossRef]
30. Carattoli, A.; Hasman, H. PlasmidFinder and In Silico pMLST: Identification and Typing of Plasmid Replicons in Whole-Genome Sequencing (WGS). *Methods Mol. Biol.* **2020**, *2075*, 285–294. [CrossRef]
31. Clausen, P.; Aarestrup, F.M.; Lund, O. Rapid and precise alignment of raw reads against redundant databases with KMA. *BMC Bioinform.* **2018**, *19*, 307. [CrossRef]
32. Larsen, M.V.; Cosentino, S.; Rasmussen, S.; Friis, C.; Hasman, H.; Marvig, R.L.; Jelsbak, L.; Sicheritz-Ponten, T.; Ussery, D.W.; Aarestrup, F.M.; et al. Multilocus sequence typing of total-genome-sequenced bacteria. *J. Clin. Microbiol.* **2012**, *50*, 1355–1361. [CrossRef]
33. Bartual, S.G.; Seifert, H.; Hippler, C.; Luzon, M.A.; Wisplinghoff, H.; Rodriguez-Valera, F. Development of a multilocus sequence typing scheme for characterization of clinical isolates of Acinetobacter baumannii. *J. Clin. Microbiol.* **2005**, *43*, 4382–4390. [CrossRef]
34. Griffiths, D.; Fawley, W.; Kachrimanidou, M.; Bowden, R.; Crook, D.W.; Fung, R.; Golubchik, T.; Harding, R.M.; Jeffery, K.J.; Jolley, K.A.; et al. Multilocus sequence typing of Clostridium difficile. *J. Clin. Microbiol.* **2010**, *48*, 770–778. [CrossRef]
35. Jaureguy, F.; Landraud, L.; Passet, V.; Diancourt, L.; Frapy, E.; Guigon, G.; Carbonnelle, E.; Lortholary, O.; Clermont, O.; Denamur, E.; et al. Phylogenetic and genomic diversity of human bacteremic Escherichia coli strains. *BMC Genom.* **2008**, *9*, 560. [CrossRef]
36. Wirth, T.; Falush, D.; Lan, R.; Colles, F.; Mensa, P.; Wieler, L.H.; Karch, H.; Reeves, P.R.; Maiden, M.C.; Ochman, H.; et al. Sex and virulence in Escherichia coli: An evolutionary perspective. *Mol. Microbiol.* **2006**, *60*, 1136–1151. [CrossRef]
37. Lemee, L.; Dhalluin, A.; Pestel-Caron, M.; Lemeland, J.F.; Pons, J.L. Multilocus sequence typing analysis of human and animal Clostridium difficile isolates of various toxigenic types. *J. Clin. Microbiol.* **2004**, *42*, 2609–2617. [CrossRef]
38. Zusman, O.; Altunin, S.; Koppel, F.; Dishon Benattar, Y.; Gedik, H.; Paul, M. Polymyxin monotherapy or in combination against carbapenem-resistant bacteria: Systematic review and meta-analysis. *J. Antimicrob. Chemother.* **2017**, *72*, 29–39. [CrossRef]
39. Shi, Q.; Han, R.; Guo, Y.; Yang, Y.; Wu, S.; Ding, L.; Zhang, R.; Yin, D.; Hu, F. Multiple Novel Ceftazidime-Avibactam-Resistant Variants of bla(KPC-2)-Positive Klebsiella pneumoniae in Two Patients. *Microbiol. Spectr.* **2022**, *10*, e0171421. [CrossRef]
40. Shields, R.K.; Chen, L.; Cheng, S.; Chavda, K.D.; Press, E.G.; Snyder, A.; Pandey, R.; Doi, Y.; Kreiswirth, B.N.; Nguyen, M.H.; et al. Emergence of Ceftazidime-Avibactam Resistance Due to Plasmid-Borne bla(KPC-3) Mutations during Treatment of Carbapenem-Resistant Klebsiella pneumoniae Infections. *Antimicrob. Agents Chemother.* **2017**, *61*, 10–1128. [CrossRef]
41. Findlay, J.; Poirel, L.; Bouvier, M.; Gaia, V.; Nordmann, P. Resistance to ceftazidime-avibactam in a KPC-2-producing Klebsiella pneumoniae caused by the extended-spectrum beta-lactamase VEB-25. *Eur. J. Clin. Microbiol. Infect. Dis.* **2023**, *42*, 639–644. [CrossRef]
42. Galani, I.; Antoniadou, A.; Karaiskos, I.; Kontopoulou, K.; Giamarellou, H.; Souli, M. Genomic characterization of a KPC-23-producing Klebsiella pneumoniae ST258 clinical isolate resistant to ceftazidime-avibactam. *Clin. Microbiol. Infect.* **2019**, *25*, 763.e5–763.e8. [CrossRef]

43. Voulgari, E.; Kotsakis, S.D.; Giannopoulou, P.; Perivolioti, E.; Tzouvelekis, L.S.; Miriagou, V. Detection in two hospitals of transferable ceftazidime-avibactam resistance in Klebsiella pneumoniae due to a novel VEB beta-lactamase variant with a Lys234Arg substitution, Greece, 2019. *Euro Surveill.* **2020**, *25*, 1900766. [CrossRef] [PubMed]
44. Evans, S.R.; Tran, T.T.T.; Hujer, A.M.; Hill, C.B.; Hujer, K.M.; Mediavilla, J.R.; Manca, C.; Domitrovic, T.N.; Perez, F.; Farmer, M.; et al. Rapid Molecular Diagnostics to Inform Empiric Use of Ceftazidime/Avibactam and Ceftolozane/Tazobactam Against Pseudomonas aeruginosa: PRIMERS IV. *Clin. Infect. Dis.* **2019**, *68*, 1823–1830. [CrossRef] [PubMed]

antibiotics

MDPI

Article

Prevalence of Carbapenemases in Carbapenem-Resistant *Acinetobacter baumannii* Isolates from the Kingdom of Bahrain

Nouf Al-Rashed [1,*], Khalid M. Bindayna [1], Mohammad Shahid [1], Nermin Kamal Saeed [2], Abdullah Darwish [3], Ronni Mol Joji [1] and Ali Al-Mahmeed [1]

1 Department of Microbiology, Immunology, and Infectious Diseases, College of Medicine & Medical Sciences, Arabian Gulf University, Manama P.O. Box 26671, Bahrain; bindayna@agu.edu.bh (K.M.B.); mohammeds@agu.edu.bh (M.S.); ronnimj@agu.edu.bh (R.M.J.); aliem@agu.edu.bh (A.A.-M.)
2 Department of Pathology, Microbiology Section, Al- Salmaniya Medical Complex, Manama P.O. Box 12, Bahrain; nhasan@health.gov.bh
3 Department of Pathology, Microbiology Section, Bahrain Defense Force Hospital, West Riffa P.O. Box 28743, Bahrain; abdulla.darwish@bdfmedical.org
* Correspondence: blueflower248@gmail.com

Abstract: Background: *Acinetobacter baumannii* is regarded as a significant cause of death in hospitals. The WHO recently added carbapenem-resistant *Acinetobacter baumannii* (CRAB) to its global pathogen priority list. There is a dearth of information on CRAB from our region. Methods: Fifty CRAB isolates were collected from four main hospitals in Bahrain for this study. Bacterial identification and antibiotic susceptibility tests were carried out using the BD Phoenix^{TM} and VITEK-2 compact, respectively. Using conventional PCR, these isolates were further screened for carbapenem resistance markers ($bla_{OXA\text{-}51}$, $bla_{OXA\text{-}23}$, $blaO_{XA\text{-}24}$, $bla_{OXA\text{-}40}$, bla_{IMP}, bla_{NDM}, bla_{VIM}, and bla_{KPC}). Results: All of the isolates were resistant to imipenem (100%), meropenem (98%), and cephalosporins (96–98%), followed by other commonly used antibiotics. All these isolates were least resistant to gentamicin (64%). The detection of resistance determinants showed that the majority harbored $bla_{OXA\text{-}51}$ (100%) and bla_{IMP} (94%), followed by $bla_{OXA\text{-}23}$ (82%), $bla_{OXA\text{-}24}$ (46%), $bla_{OXA\text{-}40}$ (14%), bla_{NDM} (6%), bla_{VIM} (2%), and bla_{KPC} (2%). Conclusion: The study isolates showed a high level of antibiotic resistance. Class D carbapenemases were more prevalent in our CRAB isolate collection. The resistance genes were found in various combinations. This study emphasizes the importance of strengthening surveillance and stringent infection control measures in clinical settings to prevent the emergence and further spread of such isolates.

Keywords: *Acinetobacter baumannii*; carbapenemases; OXA; KPC; NDM; IMP; VIM

1. Introduction

Acinetobacter baumannii (*A.baumannii*) is emerging as a significant multidrug-resistant (MDR) pathogen in hospitals, particularly in intensive care units (ICUs), and it is considered a major nosocomial pathogen causing high mortality [1,2]. The reported mortality rate is around 7.8% to 23% in hospitals and around 10% to 43% in ICUs [3]. Although there has not been any clear consensus on the associations between carbapenem-resistant *Acinetobacter baumannii* (CRAB) infections and an elevated risk of mortality [4], CRAB infections have shown a significant correlation with the length of ICU stays, elevated patient costs, and antibiotic use [4]. Moreover, it is also considered a significant pathogen causing hospital-acquired infections (HAIs) that increase the risk of the emergence of pan-drug resistance and outbreaks [5]. It usually infects human skin and wounds, especially the respiratory, gastrointestinal, and circulatory systems, causing serious infection [6]. Examples of HAIs are bacteremia, septicemia, wounds, meningitis, ventilator-associated pneumonia, and urinary tract infections [6]. Countries in the Mediterranean area have some of the highest resistance rates to carbapenems on *A. baumannii*, reaching 90%, including the Middle East, southern Europe, and North Africa [7]. The countries with the most MDR *A. baumannii* infections in the Middle East are the United Arab Emirates, Bahrain, Saudi Arabia, Palestine, and Lebanon [6]. Another epidemiological study in 2019 revealed that the resistance rates in Asia-Pacific, East Asia, Europe, North America, and Latin America were 56%, 100%, 60%, 36%, and 54%, respectively [8]. Furthermore, community-acquired pneumonia infections can also occur in several tropical countries (e.g., Asia and Australia) because of high levels of rain and humidity [6]. Owing to its significance, the World Health Organization has included CRAB in its global priority list of pathogens.

A. baumannii infections are thought to affect 1 million people worldwide each year, with 50% of those cases developing resistance to various medicines, including carbapenems [9]. Resistance is the outcome of multiple systems acting simultaneously and in unison. Specifically, these include (a) the lack and small size of outer-membrane porins whose expression can be further reduced, (b) the constitutional expression of efflux pumps (AbeABC, AbeFGH, and AbeIJK), (c) certain β-lactamases' intrinsic expression (carbapenemases, AmpC cephalosporinases, and OXA-like β-lactamases), (d) the occurrence of a 'resistance island', and (e) the ability for the horizontal acquisition of resistance determinants (OXA-23 and NDM carbapenemases, as well as aminoglycoside-modifying enzymes) [10]. Most CRAB isolates are extensively drug-resistant (XDR), indicating that they are not susceptible to antibiotic classes other than polymyxins and tigecycline [10]. Nevertheless, colistin and/or tigecycline-resistant CRAB strains are being reported more frequently [10]. As a result, a large number of clinical isolates are pan-resistant [10].

The resistance rate of *A. baumannii* to carbapenems has even reached 90% in the Middle East, southern Europe, and North Africa [7]. Most of the *A. baumannii* infections in Middle Eastern countries were reported in the United Arab Emirates, Saudi Arabia, Palestine, and Lebanon [6]. In these circumstances, it is possible that the control and treatment of CRAB will lead to new difficulties, which have sparked considerable concern in the medical community [11].

The goal of this study was to determine carbapenemase production in CRAB by identifying the specific type of *bla*-carbapenemase genes (and their prevalence) in our collection of CRAB isolates collected from four major hospitals in the Kingdom of Bahrain. Furthermore, the outcomes of gene prevalence and antibiotic susceptibility patterns were tested to discover the similarities or differences between the GCC region and the international region.

2. Results

2.1. Distribution and Antibiotic Resistance Pattern of the Isolates

The CRAB isolates used in this study were obtained from endotracheal aspirates (Number (n) = 16), blood (n = 11), urine (n = 7), wound swabs (n = 7), pus swabs (n = 4), rectal swabs (n = 3), and sputum (n = 2). These isolates showed significant resistance to imipenem (n = 50/50, 100%), meropenem and cefuroxime (n = 49/50, 98%), cefepime, cefotaxime and ceftriaxone (n = 48/50, 96%), ceftazidime (n = 45/50, 90%), amikacin (n = 21/40, 52.5%), gentamicin (n = 32/50, 64%), ampicillin/sulbactam (n = 18/29, 62.06%), ciprofloxacin (n = 46/50, 92%), levofloxacin (n = 42/50, 84%), ertapenem (n = 27/28, 96.4%), piperacillin/tazobactam (n = 41/44, 93.18%), trimethoprim/sulfamethoxazole (n = 28/47, 59.5%), minocycline (n = 11/30, 36.6%), tigecycline (n = 3/35, 8.5%), and colistin (n = 3/16, 18.75%). Details of the antibiotic resistance patterns of each isolate are shown in Figure 1A,B. The frequency of resistance of the respective antibiotics in the CRAB isolates is shown in Table 1.

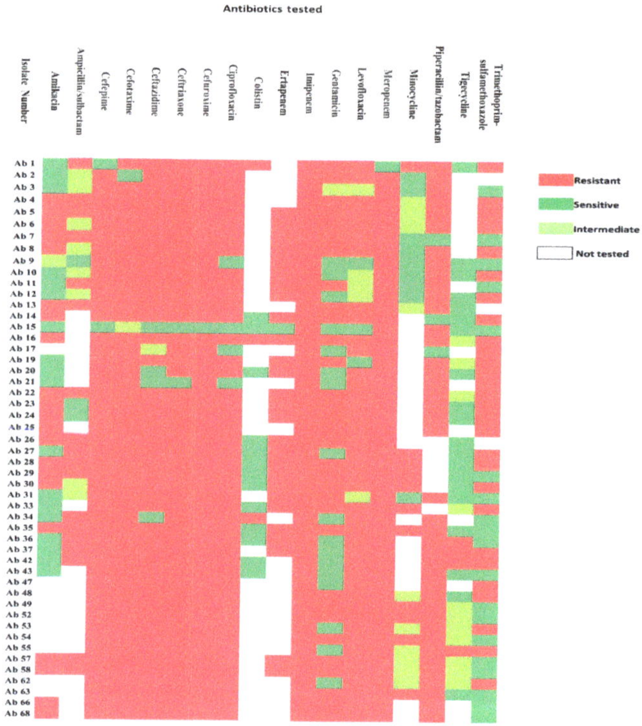

(**A**)

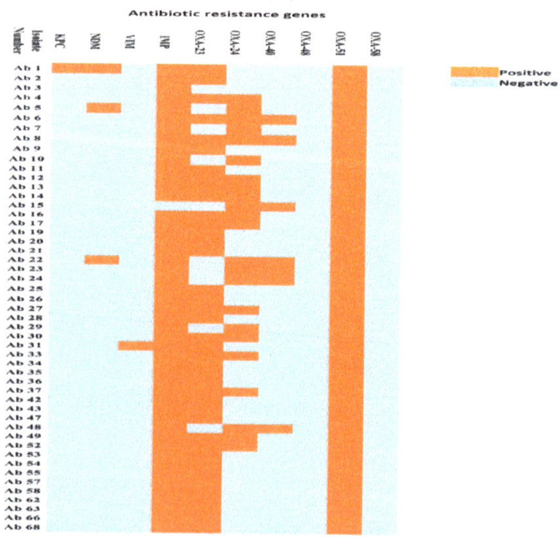

(**B**)

Figure 1. (**A**) The antibiotic resistance profile of CRAB isolates. (**B**) The presence of carbapenemases genes in CRAB isolates.

Table 1. The frequency of resistance of the respective antibiotics in the CRAB isolates.

Antibiotics	Total No. of Isolates Tested	Resistant Isolates (%)	Intermediate Isolates (%)
Amikacin	40	21 (52.5%)	1 (2.5%)
Ampicillin/sulbactam	33	22 (66.6%)	8 (24.2%)
Cefepime	50	48 (96%)	
Cefotaxin	50	48 (96%)	1 (2%)
Ceftazidime	50	45 (90%)	1 (2%)
Ceftriaxone	50	48 (96%)	
Cefuroxime	50	49 (98%)	
Ciprofloxacin	50	46 (92%)	
Colistin	18	5 (27.7%)	
Ertapenem	28	27 (96.4%)	
Imipenem	50	50 (100%)	
Gentamicin	50	32 (64%)	1 (2%)
Levofloxacin	48	42 (87.5%)	3 (6.25%)
Meropenem	50	49 (98%)	
Minocycline	30	11 (36.6%)	10 (33.3%)
Piperacillin/tazobactam	44	43 (97.7%)	
Tigecycline	35	3 (5.5%)	12 (34.2%)
Trimetoprim-sulfamethoxazole	47	28 (59.5%)	

2.2. *Carbapenemase-Encoding Genes' Detection*

Among the tested class D carbapenemases, the *bla*$_{OXA-51}$ was detected in all 50 (100%) isolates. The *bla*$_{OXA-23}$ was detected in 41 (82%) isolates, followed by *bla*$_{OXA-24}$ in 23 (46%) isolates. Seven (14%) isolates showed the presence of *bla*$_{OXA-40}$. PCR was negative for *bla*$_{OXA-48}$ and *bla*$_{OXA-58}$ in all the isolates.

Among the tested Class B carbapenemases, *bla*$_{IMP}$ was detected in 94% of the isolates (n = 47), and *bla*$_{NDM}$ was detected in 6% (n = 3) of the isolates. *bla*$_{VIM}$ and *bla*$_{KPC}$ were detected in one isolate each. Detailed results are presented in Figure 1. Various combinations of genes were noticed in our collection of CRAB isolates, ranging from as few as two genes to as many as six genes in the respective isolates (Figure 1). The majority (44%) of the isolates had a combination of three genes (*bla*$_{OXA-51}$, *bla*$_{OXA-23}$, *bla*$_{IMP}$), followed by a combination of four genes (*bla*$_{OXA-51}$, *bla*$_{OXA-23}$, *bla*$_{OXA-24}$, and *bla*$_{IMP}$) in 12 isolates (24%). The detailed results are presented in Table 2. A representative PCR gel demonstrating the respective amplicons is shown in Figure 2.

Table 2. Frequency and pattern of the combinations of carbapenem resistance genes.

Combination of Carbapenem-Resistance Genes	Number of Isolates (n = 50)
bla$_{OXA-51}$, *bla*$_{OXA-23}$, *bla*$_{OXA-24}$, *bla*$_{OXA-40}$, *bla*$_{IMP}$	2
bla$_{OXA-51}$, *bla*$_{OXA-23}$, *bla*$_{OXA-24}$, *bla*$_{IMP}$	12
bla$_{OXA-51}$, *bla*$_{OXA-23}$, *bla*$_{IMP}$	22
bla$_{OXA-51}$, *bla*$_{OXA-23}$, *bla*$_{OXA-40}$, *bla*$_{IMP}$	3
bla$_{OXA-51}$, *bla*$_{OXA-23}$,	2
bla$_{OXA-51}$, *bla*$_{OXA-24}$, *bla*$_{IMP}$	3

Table 2. *Cont.*

Combination of Carbapenem-Resistance Genes	Number of Isolates (n = 50)
bla_{OXA-51}, bla_{OXA-23}, bla_{IMP}, bla_{VIM}	1
bla_{OXA-51}, bla_{OXA-23}, bla_{OXA-24}, bla_{KPC}, bla_{IMP}, bla_{NDM}	1
bla_{OXA-51}, bla_{OXA-24}, bla_{OXA-40}, bla_{IMP}, bla_{NDM}	1
bla_{OXA-51}, bla_{OXA-24}, bla_{IMP}, bla_{NDM}	1
bla_{OXA-51}, bla_{OXA-24}, bla_{OXA-40}	1
bla_{OXA-51}, bla_{IMP}	1

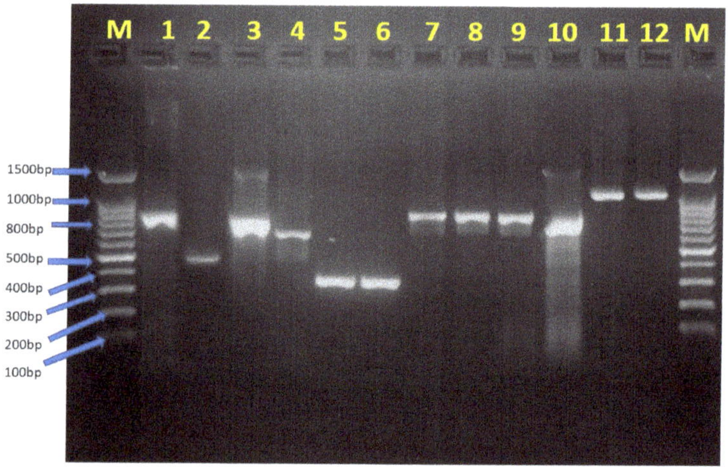

Figure 2. A representative PCR gel (1.5% agarose) showing respective *bla*-carbapenemase genes. Lane M denotes the molecular weight marker, lane 1 shows representative bla_{KPC} (881 bp), lane 2—bla_{IMP} (484 bp), lane 3—bla_{NDM} (825 bp), lane 4—bla_{VIM} (601 bp), lanes 5 and 6—bla_{OXA-51} (353 bp), lanes 7, 8, and 9—bla_{OXA-23} (821 bp), lane 10—bla_{OXA-24} (809 bp), and lanes 11 and 12—bla_{OXA-40} (1024 bp).

3. Discussion

A. baumannii is a pathogen of concern worldwide in the context of nosocomial infections owing to its multidrug resistance, often including drugs of last resort such as carbapenems [4]. This is a plausible reason why the WHO has included CRAB in its global priority list. Of the various mechanisms of carbapenem resistance in CRAB, the production of carbapenem-hydrolyzing enzymes is one of the main mechanisms of resistance [4]. These enzymes are mainly produced by the genes encoding carbapenem-hydrolyzing enzymes [4].

It is interesting to note that the Middle East was historically linked to *A. baumannii*, often known as "Iraqibacter," due to an epidemic of resistant strains among the US military during the Iraq War. Since then, hospitals around the Middle East, including those in the United Arab Emirates, Saudi Arabia, Bahrain, Palestine, and Lebanon, have isolated this bacteria [6]. *A. baumannii* has been subjected to numerous investigations testing its susceptibility to various antibiotic classes. According to a study from the holy cities of Saudi Arabia, the screening of carbapenem-resistant *A. baumannii* isolates revealed that imipenem and meropenem resistance was widespread in 81% and 84% of the strains, respectively, while the majority of the organisms were colistin- and tigecycline-susceptible [12]. Another study from Saudi Arabia concluded that eight isolates (30%) were resistant to colistin, 15 isolates (56%) were resistant to tigecycline (56%), and 24 isolates (89%) were resistant to one or more carbapenems (imipenem and meropenem] [13]. The present study showed significant resistance to imipenem, meropenem, and cephalosporins and comparatively lower resistance to minocycline, tigecycline, and colistin. Similarly, a study in China reported a high resistance rate to carbapenems and cephalosporins and a lower resistance rate to levofloxacin, minocycline, and tigecycline [14]. A two-year retrospective study from Saudi Arabia also documented that almost all isolates of *A. baumannii* were carbapenem-resistant (98%). It was interesting to note that these isolates had higher resistance to colistin (15%) when compared to tigecycline (3%) [15]. These high levels of resistance rates were caused by the overuse of imipenem and meropenem for the treatment of *A. baumannii* infection in patients [16]. As a result, recommendations for the administration of infection control procedures are required to curb the spread of these isolates in hospital settings [16].

To date, we believe that no study has determined the prevalence of carbapenemase genes from Bahrain in a relatively large cohort of CRAB isolates. Earlier, in 2015, a collaborative effort was performed in a published joint research paper incorporating *A. baumannii* isolated from the Gulf Cooperation Council (GCC) countries. Most isolates were collected from Saudi Arabia, whereas a small proportion were collected from other GCC countries (only eight isolates were gathered from Bahrain hospitals) [17]. In that study, the researchers collected a total of 117 CRAB isolates from six countries (mainly Saudi Arabia) and reported the presence of $bla_{OXA\text{-}51\text{-}type}$ in all the isolates (100%; 117/117) and that of $bla_{OXA\text{-}23\text{-}type}$ in 91% (107/117) of the isolates [17]. Cumulatively, $bla_{OXA\text{-}40\text{-}type}$ was detected in 4% (5/117) of the isolates; all five isolates positive for this gene type were from Bahrain, and none of the isolates from other GCC countries demonstrated this gene type. Among the Bahraini isolates, all eight (100%) demonstrated the presence of $bla_{OXA\text{-}51\text{-}type}$, followed by $bla_{OXA\text{-}40\text{-}type}$ (62.5%), and three isolates (38%; 3/8) showed $bla_{OXA\text{-}23\text{-}type}$ [17]. The authors also reported the non-detection of $bla_{OXA\text{-}58}$, bla_{KPC}, and metallo-beta-lactamases (MBLs) like bla_{IMP} and bla_{VIM} [17].

In another report published based on a study in Bahrain in 2009, where eight isolates were again molecularly tested for these carbapenemase genes [18], the most prevalent reported gene was $bla_{OXA\text{-}40\text{-}like}$ (in five isolates), followed by $bla_{OXA\text{-}23}$ (two isolates) and $bla_{OXA\text{-}58}$ (one isolate) [18].

In the current study, $bla_{OXA\text{-}51}$, $bla_{OXA\text{-}23}$, $bla_{OXA\text{-}24}$, and bla_{IMP} were the most commonly detected carbapenemase-producing genes, occurring at frequencies of 100%, 82%, 46%, and 94%, respectively. In contrast to the previous reports, our collection of CRAB isolates also showed the presence of bla_{VIM}, bla_{NDM}, bla_{KPC}, and $bla_{OXA\text{-}40}$, though with lesser frequency. None of our isolates showed the presence of $bla_{OXA\text{-}48}$ or $bla_{OXA\text{-}58}$. Even though it is too early to speculate on the present context due to the small number of isolates tested previously, it looks as if the molecular epidemiology in Bahrain has changed over the years, with the predominant gene now being $bla_{OXA\text{-}23}$, which was comparatively less prevalent earlier. The $bla_{OXA\text{-}40}$ gene has become less prevalent, being the predominant gene reported in previous studies. It is also alarming to note the presence of a combination of carbapenem-resistance genes in some isolates at a level as high as six genes. MBLs and bla_{KPC} were rarely reported in *A. baumannii* isolates, except for bla_{IMP}. However, in our isolates, we found the presence of bla_{IMP} in a significantly higher percentage (94%), which is also alarming. It was noticed that there was no correlation between the combinations of carbapenemase genes and the antibiotic resistance pattern. The CRAB isolates were highly resistant to all carbapenems and most cephalosporins with lower resistance to other antibiotics.

The $bla_{OXA\text{-}51}$ is generally found in all *A. baumannii* isolates, being either carbapenem-resistant or carbapenem-sensitive isolates [19–21]. This gene is not associated with resistance unless insertion sequences (*ISAbaI*) upstream of $bla_{OXA\text{-}51}$ are involved, causing over-expression leading to carbapenem resistance, especially to imipenem [21,22]. Therefore, it is recommended as an excellent marker for species identification but not as a resistance marker [22–25].

On the other hand, $bla_{OXA\text{-}23}$ is a significant cause of carbapenem resistance in *A. baumannii* [19,21,22]. It has been reported as a prevalent gene in various studies published in several countries, including Saudi Arabia and Iran [19,21]. In contrast to this, a few other international studies have observed the presence of bla_{OXA-23} at a lower frequency, as reported in Bosnia, Poland, and Croatia [21]. The bla_{OXA-24} gene is also reported as a common gene, albeit at variable percentages [19,22,23]. On the Arabian Peninsula, another study from Egypt investigated the prevalence of carbapenemase genes in 40 CRAB isolates [26]. The bla_{OXA-51} gene was amplified in all isolates, whereas bla_{OXA-23}, bla_{OXA-24}, and bla_{OXA-58} were present in 50%, 7.5%, and 5% of the isolates. All these isolates lacked bla_{KPC} or MBLs [26].

In a study conducted in Iran in 2015, Azizi O et al. observed that bla_{OXA-51} and bla_{OXA-23} were present in all isolates but were negative for bla_{OXA-58} [19]. In South Africa, Lowings M. et al. reported two genes (bla_{OXA-51} and bla_{OXA-23}) among 100 MDR *A. baumannii* isolates (99 and 77%, respectively) [25]. The other genes, such as bla_{OXA-24}, bla_{OXA-58}, bla_{KPC}, and MBLs, were negative [25]. Various other international studies outside of the GCC region also reported the presence of these genes, albeit with varying frequencies [24,27]. However, it is interesting to note that many of these studies reported the absence of genes such as bla_{OXA-24}, bla_{OXA-58}, bla_{IMP}, bla_{VIM}, and bla_{KPC} [27].

Alarmingly, a significant proportion of the isolates in our collection also demonstrated concomitant resistance to fluoroquinolones and the aminoglycoside group of antibiotics. For other last-resort antibiotics such as tigecycline and colistin, even though the isolates demonstrated a lower frequency of resistance, the appearance of resistance is quite alarming.

This study has a few limitations. One is that the analysis of resistance determinants using molecular methods was limited to carbapenemases in CRAB isolates and did not include the details of ESBL and other antibiotic resistance mechanisms. In addition, sequencing was not performed to search for gene mutations. However, to the best of our knowledge, this is the first report describing the prevalence (and molecular characterization) of CRAB isolates in a relatively large cohort from the Kingdom of Bahrain.

4. Materials and Methods

4.1. Bacterial Isolates and Hospital Setting

From February 2021 to June 2022, 50 random, nonrepetitive CRAB isolates were collected from the microbiology labs of four different hospitals (Al-Salmaniya Medical Complex, Bahrain Defense Force Hospital, King Hamad University Hospital, and Bahrain Specialist Hospital) in the Kingdom of Bahrain. These isolates were cultured from specimens such as endotracheal aspirates, urine, sputum, blood cultures, wounds, pus, and rectal swabs. The isolates obtained from the lab were preserved in glycerol milk at certain volumes (3 mL and 4 mL) with 13 mL of deionized water and stored at −80 °C until further testing [28].

4.2. Bacterial Identification and Antibiotic Susceptibility Testing

The bacterial species-level identification and antibiotic susceptibility testing of the isolates were performed with automated microbiological systems (Vitek2 automated system) at the Bahrain Defense Force Hospital and Bahrain Specialist Hospital and a BD Phoenix™ automated system at the Al-Salmaniya Medical Complex and King Hamad University Hospital. Only the isolates that were identified as *A. baumannii* resistant to carbapenems were included for further molecular analysis. As per each hospital's antibiotic policies, the isolates were tested against certain antibiotics. The tested and non-tested antibiotics are presented in Figure 1A.

4.3. Amplification of Carbapenemases Genes via Polymerase Chain Reaction

For carbapenemase gene detection, the DNA of the bacterial strains was extracted from the CRAB pure culture using the boiling method [29]. The PCR reactions were carried out in a total volume of 25 µL, consisting of 12.5 µL of PCR Master Mix, 9 µL of DNase/RNase-free water, 0.5 µL each of forward and reverse primer, and 2.5 µL of DNA template. Each primer specific for the carbapenemase genes (Class A: bla_{KPC}; Class B: bla_{IMP}, bla_{NDM}, and

bla_{VIM}; Class D: $bla_{OXA\text{-}23}$, $bla_{OXA\text{-}24}$, $bla_{OXA\text{-}40}$, $bla_{OXA\text{-}48}$, $bla_{OXA\text{-}51}$, and $bla_{OXA\text{-}58}$) had a specific thermal cycle that was optimized separately. The amplicons were detected via 1.5% gel electrophoresis, and the bands were visualized under UV illumination [22]. The positive quality control strains used were multidrug-resistant *A. baumannii* ATCC 19606 and *Klebsiella pneumoniae*. The specific primers and the cycling conditions used in the study are shown in Table 3.

Table 3. List of carbapenemase-gene-specific primers used in this study.

Genes Targeted	Primer Sequence (5′→3′)	Amplicon Size (bp)	Reference
KPC	F-ATGTCACTGTATCGCCGTCT R-TTACTGCCCGTTGACGCCCA	881	[20]
VIM	F-ATTCCGGTCGG(A=G) GAGGTCCG R-TGTGCTKGAGCAAKTCYAGACCG	601	[20]
NDM	F-GGCCGTATGAGTGATTGC R-GAAGCTGAGCACCGCATTAG	825	[20]
IMP	F-CGGCC(G=T) CAGGAG(A=C) G(G-T) CTTT R-AACCAGTTTTGC(C=T) TTAC(C=T) AT	484	[20]
OXA-23	F-ATGAATAAATATTTTACTTG RTTAAATAATATTCAGCTGTT	821	[20]
OXA-24	F-ATACTTCCTATATTCAGCAT R-GATTCCAAGATTTCTAGCG	809	[20]
OXA-40	F-GTACTAATCAAAGTTGTGAA R-TTCCCCTAACATGAATTTGT	1024	[30]
OXA-48	F-GCTTGATCGCCCTCGATT R-GATTTGCTCCGTGGCCGAAA	281	[20]
OXA-51	F-TAATGCTTTGATCGGCCTTC R-TGGATTGCACTTCATCTTGG	353	[20]
OXA-58	F-ATGAAATTATTAAAAATATTGAGT R-ATAAATAATGAAAAACACCCAA	840	[20]

5. Conclusions

This study provides a clear picture of the currently prevalent bla-carbapenemases in the Kingdom of Bahrain. Oxacillinases (Class D) were the predominant carbapenemases; the most common genes detected were $bla_{OXA\text{-}51}$ and $bla_{OXA\text{-}23}$. From Class B, bla_{IMP} was also detected at a significantly higher percentage. The presence of other Class B genes (such as bla_{NDM} and bla_{VIM}) and Class A genes (bla_{KPC}), though in smaller percentages, is quite alarming. The rate of resistance to most antibiotics is high in our region. These results emphasize the significance of rational antibiotic therapy and ongoing stringent surveillance and infection control strategies to successfully curb the spread of these clinical strains.

Author Contributions: N.A.-R.: conceptualization, preliminary draft, collection of isolates, experimentation including molecular experiments, and initial analysis; K.M.B.: conceptualization, evaluation, interpretation of results, and review, editing, and approval of final draft; M.S.: conceptualization, evaluation, interpretation of results, and review, editing and approval of final draft; N.K.S.: provided clinical isolates, identified them and performed antibiotic susceptibility testing on automated systems; A.D.: provided clinical isolates, identified them and performed antibiotic susceptibility testing on automated systems; R.M.J.: edited the draft; A.A.-M.: helped with the practical work, especially the molecular experiments. All authors have read and agreed to the published version of the manuscript.

Funding: An internal grant was provided by the Arabian Gulf University, Bahrain (Student Project No. E25-P1-01/20), awarded to Nouf Al-Rashed towards a Ph.D. on the Molecular Medicine Program at the Arabian Gulf University.

Institutional Review Board Statement: The study was approved by the institutional Research and Ethics Committee of the Arabian Gulf University, approval No. E25-P1-01/20, and by the Ministry of Health, Kingdom of Bahrain (AURS/ 360/2020).

Informed Consent Statement: Not applicable.

Data Availability Statement: We confirm that all the data are presented in this article.

Acknowledgments: The authors would like to thank all the technical staff of the hospital laboratories that participated in this study.

Conflicts of Interest: The authors have no conflicts of interest.

References

1. Howard, A.; O'Donoghue, M.; Feeney, A.; Sleator, R.D. Acinetobacter baumannii: An emerging opportunistic pathogen. *Virulence* **2012**, *3*, 243–250. [CrossRef] [PubMed]
2. Vijayakumar, S.; Biswas, I.; Veeraraghavan, B. Accurate identification of clinically important *Acinetobacter* spp.: An update. *Future Sci. OA* **2019**, *5*, FSO395. [CrossRef] [PubMed]
3. Zhang, Y.; Ding, F.; Luo, Y.; Fan, B.; Tao, Z.; Li, Y.; Gu, D. Distribution pattern of carbapenemases and solitary contribution to resistance in clinical strains of Acinetobacter baumannii. *Ann. Palliat. Med.* **2021**, *10*, 9184–9191. [CrossRef]
4. Ejaz, H.; Ahmad, M.; Younas, S.; Junaid, K.; Abosalif, K.O.A.; Abdalla, A.E.; Alameen, A.A.M.; Elamir, M.Y.M.; Bukhari, S.N.A.; Ahmad, N.; et al. Molecular Epidemiology of Extensively-Drug Resistant Acinetobacter baumannii Sequence Type 2 Co-Harboring bla (NDM) and bla (OXA) From Clinical Origin. *Infect. Drug Resist.* **2021**, *14*, 1931–1939. [CrossRef]
5. Fournier, P.E.; Richet, H. The epidemiology and control of Acinetobacter baumannii in health care facilities. *Clin. Infect. Dis.* **2006**, *42*, 692–699. [CrossRef] [PubMed]
6. Almasaudi, S.B. Acinetobacter spp. as nosocomial pathogens: Epidemiology and resistance features. *Saudi J. Biol. Sci.* **2018**, *25*, 586–596. [CrossRef]
7. Ma, C.; McClean, S. Mapping Global Prevalence of Acinetobacter baumannii and Recent Vaccine Development to Tackle It. *Vaccines* **2021**, *9*, 570. [CrossRef]
8. Gales, A.C.; Seifert, H.; Gur, D.; Castanheira, M.; Jones, R.N.; Sader, H.S. Antimicrobial Susceptibility of Acinetobacter calcoaceticus-Acinetobacter baumannii Complex and Stenotrophomonas maltophilia Clinical Isolates: Results From the SENTRY Antimicrobial Surveillance Program (1997-2016). *Open Forum Infect. Dis.* **2019**, *6* (Suppl. 1), S34–S46. [CrossRef]
9. Spellberg, B.; Rex, J.H. The value of single-pathogen antibacterial agents. *Nat. Rev. Drug Discov.* **2013**, *12*, 963. [CrossRef]
10. Wong, D.; Nielsen, T.B.; Bonomo, R.A.; Pantapalangkoor, P.; Luna, B.; Spellberg, B. Clinical and Pathophysiological Overview of Acinetobacter Infections: A Century of Challenges. *Clin. Microbiol. Rev.* **2017**, *30*, 409–447. [CrossRef]
11. Jiang, Y.; Ding, Y.; Wei, Y.; Jian, C.; Liu, J.; Zeng, Z. Carbapenem-resistant Acinetobacter baumannii: A challenge in the intensive care unit. *Front. Microbiol.* **2022**, 13. [CrossRef]
12. Al-Sultan, A.A. Prevalence of High-Risk Antibiotic Resistant Acinetobacter baumannii in the Holy Cities of Makkah and Al-Madinah. *Open Microbiol. J.* **2021**, *15*, 145–151. [CrossRef]
13. Al-Agamy, M.H.; Jeannot, K.; El-Mahdy, T.S.; Shibl, A.M.; Kattan, W.; Plésiat, P.; Courvalin, P. First detection of GES-5 carbapenemase-producing Acinetobacter baumannii isolate. *Microb. Drug Resist.* **2017**, *23*, 556–562. [CrossRef] [PubMed]
14. Zhu, Y.; Zhang, X.; Wang, Y.; Tao, Y.; Shao, X.; Li, Y.; Li, W. Insight into carbapenem resistance and virulence of Acinetobacter baumannii from a children's medical centre in eastern China. *Ann. Clin. Microbiol. Antimicrob.* **2022**, *21*, 47. [CrossRef]
15. Hafiz, T.A.; Alghamdi, S.S.; Mubaraki, M.A.; Alghamdi, S.S.M.; Alothaybi, A.; Aldawood, E.; Alotaibi, F. A two-year retrospective study of multidrug-resistant Acinetobacter baumannii respiratory infections in critically Ill patients: Clinical and microbiological findings. *J. Infect. Public Health* **2023**, *16*, 313–319. [CrossRef] [PubMed]
16. Al-Obeid, S.; Jabri, L.; Al-Agamy, M.; Al-Omari, A.; Shibl, A. Epidemiology of extensive drug resistant Acinetobacter baumannii (XDRAB) at Security Forces Hospital (SFH) in Kingdom of Saudi Arabia (KSA). *J. Chemother.* **2015**, *27*, 156–162. [CrossRef] [PubMed]
17. Zowawi, H.M.; Sartor, A.L.; Sidjabat, H.E.; Balkhy, H.H.; Walsh, T.R.; Al Johani, S.M.; AlJindan, R.Y.; Alfaresi, M.; Ibrahim, E.; Al-Jardani, A.; et al. Molecular epidemiology of carbapenem-resistant Acinetobacter baumannii isolates in the Gulf Cooperation Council States: Dominance of OXA-23-type producers. *J. Clin. Microbiol.* **2015**, *53*, 896–903. [CrossRef]
18. Mugnier, P.D.; Bindayna, K.M.; Poirel, L.; Nordmann, P. Diversity of plasmid-mediated carbapenem-hydrolysing oxacillinases among carbapenem-resistant Acinetobacter baumannii isolates from Kingdom of Bahrain. *J. Antimicrob. Chemother.* **2009**, *63*, 1071–1073. [CrossRef]
19. Azizi, O.; Shakibaie, M.R.; Modarresi, F.; Shahcheraghi, F. Molecular Detection of Class-D OXA Carbapenemase Genes in Biofilm and Non-Biofilm Forming Clinical Isolates of Acinetobacter baumannii. *Jundishapur. J. Microbiol.* **2015**, *8*, e21042. [CrossRef]
20. Soudeiha, M.A.H.; Dahdouh, E.A.; Azar, E.; Sarkis, D.K.; Daoud, Z. In vitro Evaluation of the Colistin-Carbapenem Combination in Clinical Isolates of A. baumannii Using the Checkerboard, Etest, and Time-Kill Curve Techniques. *Front. Cell. Infect. Microbiol.* **2017**, *7*, 209. [CrossRef]

21. Ibrahimagic, A.; Kamberovic, F.; Uzunovic, S.; Bedenic, B.; Idrizovic, E. Molecular characteristics and antibiotic resistance of Acinetobacter baumanniibeta-lactamase-producing isolates, a predominance of intrinsic blaOXA-51, and detection of TEM and CTX-M genes. *Turk. J. Med. Sci.* **2017**, *47*, 715–720. [CrossRef] [PubMed]
22. Amudhan, S.M.; Sekar, U.; Arunagiri, K.; Sekar, B. OXA beta-lactamase-mediated carbapenem resistance in Acinetobacter baumannii. *Indian J. Med. Microbiol.* **2011**, *29*, 269–274. [CrossRef] [PubMed]
23. Grisold, A.J.; Luxner, J.; Bedenic, B.; Diab-Elschahawi, M.; Berktold, M.; Wechsler-Fordos, A.; Zarfel, G.E. Diversity of Oxacillinases and Sequence Types in Carbapenem-Resistant Acinetobacter baumannii from Austria. *Int. J. Environ. Res. Public Health* **2021**, *18*, 2171. [CrossRef] [PubMed]
24. Wang, T.H.; Leu, Y.S.; Wang, N.Y.; Liu, C.P.; Yan, T.R. Prevalence of different carbapenemase genes among carbapenem-resistant Acinetobacter baumannii blood isolates in Taiwan. *Antimicrob. Resist. Infect. Control* **2018**, *7*, 123. [CrossRef]
25. Lowings, M.; Ehlers, M.M.; Dreyer, A.W.; Kock, M.M. High prevalence of oxacillinases in clinical multidrug-resistant Acinetobacter baumannii isolates from the Tshwane region, South Africa—An update. *BMC Infect. Dis.* **2015**, *15*, 521. [CrossRef]
26. Al-Agamy, M.H.; Khalaf, N.G.; Tawfick, M.M.; Shibl, A.M.; El Kholy, A. Molecular characterization of carbapenem-insensitive Acinetobacter baumannii in Egypt. *Int. J. Infect. Dis.* **2014**, *22*, 49–54. [CrossRef]
27. Xiao, S.Z.; Chu, H.Q.; Han, L.Z.; Zhang, Z.M.; Li, B.; Zhao, L.; Xu, L. Resistant mechanisms and molecular epidemiology of imipenem-resistant Acinetobacter baumannii. *Mol. Med. Rep.* **2016**, *14*, 2483–2488. [CrossRef]
28. Cody, W.L.; Wilson, J.W.; Hendrixson, D.R.; McIver, K.S.; Hagman, K.E.; Ott, C.M.; Nickerson, C.A.; Schurr, M.J. Skim milk enhances the preservation of thawed -80 degrees C bacterial stocks. *J. Microbiol. Methods* **2008**, *75*, 135–138. [CrossRef]
29. Shahid, M.; Sobia, F.; Singh, A.; Khan, H.M. Concurrent occurrence of blaampC families and blaCTX-M genogroups and association with mobile genetic elements ISEcp1, IS26, ISCR1, and sul1-type class 1 integrons in Escherichia coli and Klebsiella pneumoniae isolates originating from India. *J. Clin. Microbiol.* **2012**, *50*, 1779–1782. [CrossRef]
30. Charfi-Kessis, K.; Mansour, W.; Ben Haj Khalifa, A.; Mastouri, M.; Nordmann, P.; Aouni, M.; Poirel, L. Multidrug-resistant Acinetobacter baumannii strains carrying the bla(OxA-23) and the bla(GES-11) genes in a neonatology center in Tunisia. *Microb. Pathog.* **2014**, *74*, 20–24. [CrossRef]

antibiotics

MDPI

Article

Evaluation of Five Host Inflammatory Biomarkers in Early Diagnosis of Ventilator-Associated Pneumonia in Critically Ill Children: A Prospective Single Center Cohort Study

Maria Sdougka [1], Maria Simitsopoulou [2], Elena Volakli [1], Asimina Violaki [1], Vivian Georgopoulou [3], Argiro Ftergioti [2], Emmanuel Roilides [2] and Elias Iosifidis [2,*]

[1] Pediatric Intensive Care Unit, Hippokration General Hospital, 54942 Thessaloniki, Greece
[2] Infectious Disease Unit, 3rd Department of Pediatrics, School of Medicine, Faculty of Health Sciences, Hippokration General Hospital, 54942 Thessaloniki, Greece
[3] Medical Imaging Department, Hippokration General Hospital, 54942 Thessaloniki, Greece
* Correspondence: iosifidish@auth.gr; Tel.: +30-2310-892486; Fax: +30-2310-992981

Abstract: Background: Early diagnosis of ventilator-associated pneumonia (VAP) remains a challenge due to subjective clinical criteria and the low discriminative power of diagnostic tests. We assessed whether rapid molecular diagnostics in combination with Clinically Pulmonary Index Score (CPIS) scoring, microbiological surveillance and biomarker measurements of PTX-3, SP-D, s-TREM, PTX-3, IL-1β and IL-8 in the blood or lung could improve the accuracy of VAP diagnosis and follow-up in critically ill children. **Methods**: A prospective pragmatic study in a Pediatric Intensive Care Unit (PICU) was conducted on ventilated critically ill children divided into two groups: high and low suspicion of VAP according to modified Clinically Pulmonary Index Score (mCPIS). Blood and bronchial samples were collected on days 1, 3, 6 and 12 after event onset. Rapid diagnostics were used for pathogen identification and ELISA for PTX-3, SP-D, s-TREM, IL-1β and IL-8 measurements. **Results:** Among 20 enrolled patients, 12 had a high suspicion (mCPIS > 6), and 8 had a low suspicion of VAP (mCPIS < 6); 65% were male; and 35% had chronic disease. IL-1β levels at day 1 correlated significantly with the number of mechanical ventilation days ($r_s = 0.67$, $p < 0.001$) and the PICU stay ($r = 0.66$; $p < 0.002$). No significant differences were found in the levels of the other biomarkers between the two groups. Mortality was recorded in two patients with high VAP suspicion. **Conclusions:** PTX-3, SP-D, s-TREM, IL-1β and IL-8 biomarkers could not discriminate patients with a high or low suspicion of VAP diagnosis.

Keywords: ventilator-associated pneumonia; critically ill children; biomarkers

1. Introduction

Ventilator-associated pneumonia (VAP) is the second most common hospital-acquired infection after bloodstream infections in critically ill children [1]. Pneumonia development leads to longer duration of mechanical ventilation, prolonged hospital stay and broad-spectrum antibiotic use, and it contributes to high morbidity and mortality rates [2,3]. In addition, in critically ill children hospitalized with pneumonia, those with VAP have worse outcomes than those with severe community-acquired pneumonia [4].

Several pediatric studies report that the frequency of VAP in the Pediatric Intensive Care Units (PICUs) worldwide is in the range of 2 to 35%. Such significant variation is attributed to, among other things, differences in case definition, sampling procedure and diagnostic method [5,6]. The most recent National Health Safety Network (NHSN) module published by the Centers for Disease Control and Prevention on definitions specific to VAP underlines that early-onset VAP is suspected when microorganism invasion of the lower respiratory tract occurs on more than two consecutive calendar days from the date of event in patients on mechanical ventilator support [7]. However, due to the lack of universally employed diagnostic algorithms, an accurate VAP diagnosis remains a great challenge, hampering timely administration of antibiotic regimens, clear assessment of existing VAP burden in PICUs and development of effective preventive strategies [8].

The use of clinical scores such as the Clinical Pulmonary Infection Score (CPIS) (fever, leukocytosis, bronchial aspirates, oxygenation and radiographic pulmonary infiltrates) and microbiological tests are insufficient to discriminate VAP from other non-infectious conditions. This is due to the subjective assessment of clinical criteria, interobserver variability, inherently low specificity or sensitivity as well as delayed differential diagnosis ranging from 48 to 72 h [9]. Thus, in conjunction with clinical scoring for suspected VAP, the use of molecular diagnostic platforms for the rapid identification of the most common respiratory pathogens, combined with the use of biomarkers of infection employing non-invasive sampling procedures, needs to be explored to determine their clinical value in early diagnosis of VAP in critically ill children.

Accurate and rapid identification of true lung infection for targeted antibiotic treatment is the most important attribute that underscores the rationale for using biomarkers in clinical practice. Although the value and net health benefit for a number of biomarkers in VAP diagnosis has been investigated, the results of clinical studies remain contradictory. For example, the diagnostic value of single measurements performed for PCT (procalcitonin), a prohormone released in serum in response to inflammation, CRP (C-reactive Protein), an acute-phase protein and soluble triggering receptor expressed on myeloid cells and s-TREM biomarker, a glycoprotein member of the immunoglobulin family up-regulated in the presence of pathogens, has not been demonstrated as they cannot discriminate between suspected VAP and non-VAP cases [10–12]. SP-D (surfactant protein D, expressed by type II alveolar cells and involved in innate immunity on all mucosal surfaces, was found to be a bacterial species-specific differentiating factor in children with VAP. In VAP diagnosis, it was the most sensitive to PTX-3 (pentraxin-3), a member of the pentraxin subfamily correlated with lung injury severity in acute respiratory syndromes [13,14].

However, studies have shown that combining results from measurements of multiple biomarkers may provide significant discriminative power between infectious and non-infectious causes of inflammatory responses [15]. Systematic analyses concluded that a panel of biomarkers measured at different time points for grasping biomarker dynamics, used in conjunction with clinical diagnosis and scoring systems, may significantly improve early VAP diagnosis and antibiotic therapy [16,17].

Most of these biomarkers as well as cytokines such as IL-1β (interleukin-1-beta) and IL-8 (interleukin-8) have been investigated mostly in serum and bronchoalveolar lavage (BAL) samples to evaluate their association with VAP in adult patients. In current clinical practice, both CRP and PCT measurements are used in combination with clinical and microbiological criteria [17,18]. However, according to the most recent clinical guidelines for VAP diagnosis in adults, the initiation of antibiotic therapy should be driven by clinical criteria alone without taking into account CRP or PCT [19].

Unfortunately, there are even fewer data on the role of biomarkers for VAP diagnosis in children. The biomarkers s-TREM and PTX-3 have been investigated in only four pediatric studies with controversial results regarding their diagnostic accuracy [13,20–22], whereas no studies to date exist for the clinical value of IL-1β and IL-8 in early diagnosis of VAP in critically ill children.

In this study we assess whether using a polymerase chain reaction (PCR)-based rapid diagnostic tool to detect VAP-associated pathogens and resistance genes in the lower respiratory tract, in combination with CPIS scoring, microbiological tests and the levels of PTX-3, SP-D, s-TREM, IL-1β, and IL-8 in serum and/or lower respiratory tract aspirate, could improve the accuracy of VAP diagnosis and follow-up in critically-ill children.

2. Results

Characteristics of the patients: Over the 16-month study, 27 children were screened and 20 (74%) were included in the study. According to the mCPIS, the high VAP suspicion group (mCPIS > 6) was made up of 12 children and the low VAP suspicion group (mCPIS < 6) consisted of 8 children. Of the total population, 65% were male. The median age was 24.5 (6–141) months in the high suspicion group and 129 (28–184) months in low-suspicion group. Thirty five percent had chronic disease and 40% acute illness (Table 1). All children were on mechanical ventilation and were treated with antibiotics on day 1 of the study. Analysis of clinical characteristics presented in Table 1 showed no significant differences between high and low VAP suspicion groups.

Table 1. Clinical characteristics of the study population.

	Total Population n = 20	Patient Groups with VAP [1] Suspicion High (n = 12)	Low (n = 8)	*p* Value
sex, male, n (%)	13 (65)	9 (75)	5 (63)	
Age [2], mo	93 (6–184)	24.5 (6–141)	129 (28–184)	
underlying disease				
trauma, n (%)	3 (15)	3 (25)	0.0	
surgery, n (%)	2 (10)	2 (17)	0.0	
chronic disease *, n (%)	7 (35)	3 (25)	4 (50)	
acute illness, n (%)	8 (40)	4 (33.3)	4 (50)	
PRISM [3] III score [2]	11 (5–27)	13 (5–27)	10.5 (5–19)	0.443 [a]
body temperature, (°C) [6]	37.7 (0.97)	37.9 (1.07)	37.3 (0.64)	
vasopressors/shock, n (%)	14 (70)	10 (83)	5 (63)	
transfusions, n (%)	7 (35)	5 (42)	2 (25)	
CVC [7], n (%)	20 (100)	12 (100)	8 (100)	
nasogastric tube, n (%)	20 (100)	12 (100)	8 (100)	
folley, n (%)	19 (95)	11 (92)	8 (100)	
enteral, n (%)	18 (90)	10 (83)	8 (100)	
antibiotics, n (%)	20 (100)	12 (100)	8 (100)	
parenteral nutrition, n (%)	2 (10)	2 (17)	0.0	
time to enrollment [2], d	6 (4–29)	6 (4–29)	7 (2–26)	0.6 [a]
mCPIS [2,5]	6.5 (3–9)	7.25 (5–9)	4.25 (3–8)	<0.01 [b]
positive culture, n (%)	4 (20)	0.0	4 (100)	
time on mechanical ventilation [2], d	29 (5–62)	21.5 (8–62)	32 (5–43)	0.716 [a]
length of PICU stay [2,4], d	31.5 (7–62)	26.5 (7–62)	35.5 (7–55)	0.967 [a]
length of hospital stay [2], d	56.5 (6–181)	56.5 (7–181)	65 (6–155)	0.53 [a]
death in PICU, n (%)	1 (5)	1 (8)	0.0	
mortality, n (%)	2 (10)	2 (17)	0.0	0.49

[1] VAP: Ventilator-Associated Pneumonia, [2] median, range, [3] PRISM: Pediatric Risk of Mortality, [4] PICU: Pediatric Intensive Care Unit, [5] mCPIS: modified Clinical Pulmonary Infection Score [6] mean ± standard deviation, [7] CVC: Central Venous Catheter. [a] Mann-Whitney U test, [b] Student's *t* test, * GABA transaminase deficiency, pantothenate kinase-associated neurodegeneration, Batten syndrome, cerebral palsy, epileptic encephalopathy, Noonan syndrome, Leigh syndrome.

Molecular and microbiological assessment: Rapid molecular diagnostics conducted on bronchial secretions of patients obtained on day 1 identified *Staphylococcus aureus* in one patient and *Acinetobacter baumannii* in three others, all of whom were in the low VAP suspicion group. Blood cultures during the four timepoints of the study remained negative. Two non-colonized patients in the low VAP suspicion group, with declining CRP levels on day 6 (91 and 24 mg/L), developed sepsis on day 12 of the study, which increased CRP levels to 278 mg/L. These two patients were therefore excluded from the data analysis of the CRP biomarker on day 12 of the study (Figure 1, panel C).

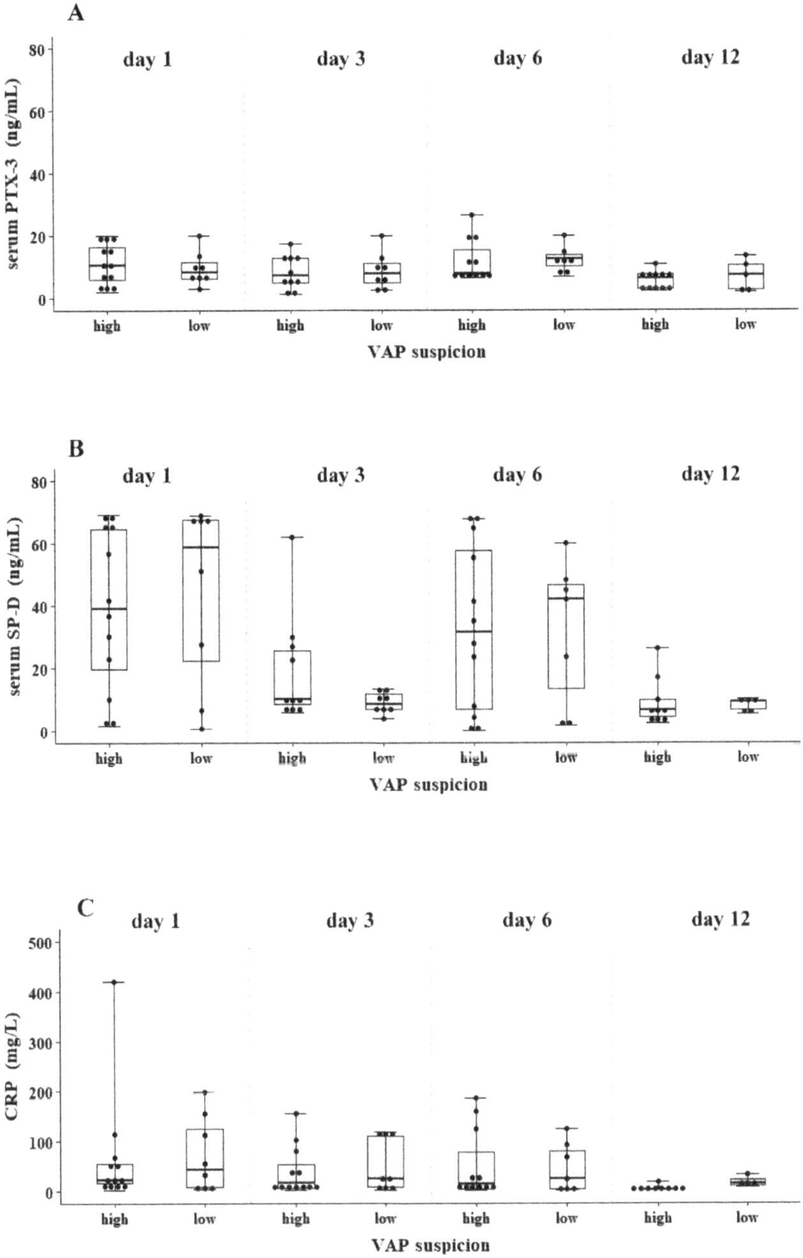

Figure 1. Serum PTX-3, SP-D and CRP levels of critically ill children with VAP suspicion. Box (interquartile) and whisker (range) plots show the concentration of PTX-3 (ng/mL; panel (**A**)), SP-D (ng/mL; panel (**B**)) and CRP (mg/L; panel (**C**)) in blood at days 1, 3, 6 and 12 from patients with mechanical ventilation. The patients with VAP suspicion were assigned into two groups based on CPIS scores: high (CPIS > 6) and low (CPIS < 6). Statistically significant differences between groups were examined using the non-parametric ANOVA Kruskal–Wallis with Dunn's multiple comparisons test.

Biomarker levels in bronchial secretions and serum: No significant differences were found in PTX-3, SP-D, s-TREM, IL-1β and IL-8 levels between the high and low VAP suspicion groups. In serum, the median levels of PTX-3, SP-D and CRP levels at the four timepoints in the high VAP group were 6–10 ng/mL, 6–39 ng/mL and 2–30 mg/L compared to 7–8 ng/mL, 8.3–58 ng/mL and 15–43 mg/L in the low VAP group, respectively (Figure 1, panels A–C). In bronchial aspirates, the levels of PTX-3, SP-D, s-TREM, IL-1β and IL-8 at days 3 and 6 were also similar in both VAP groups (Figure 2, panels A–D).

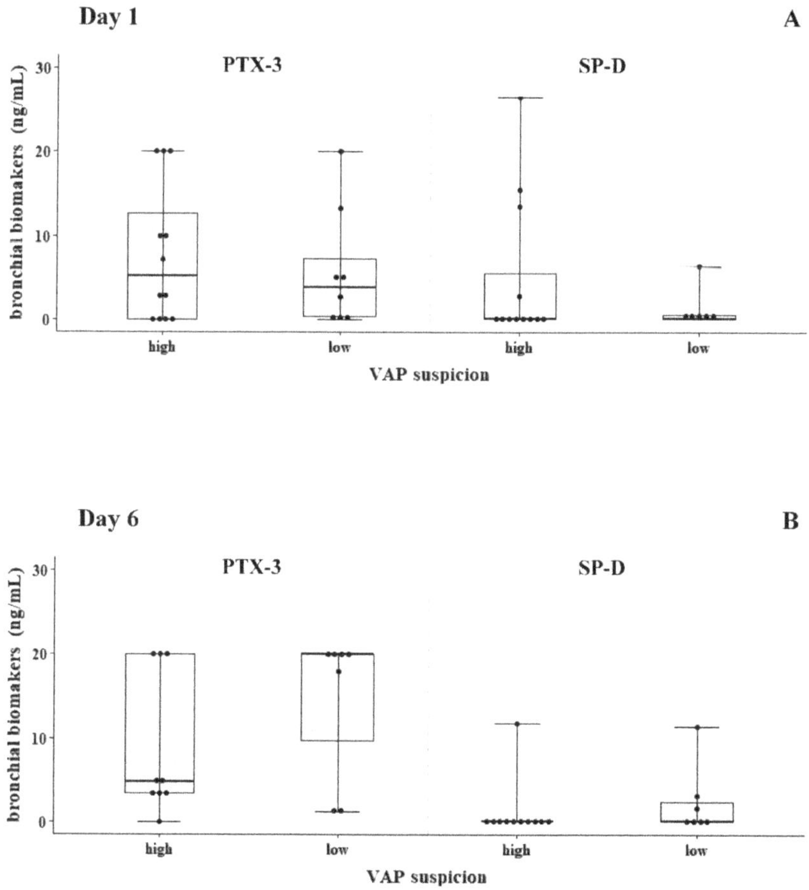

Figure 2. *Cont.*

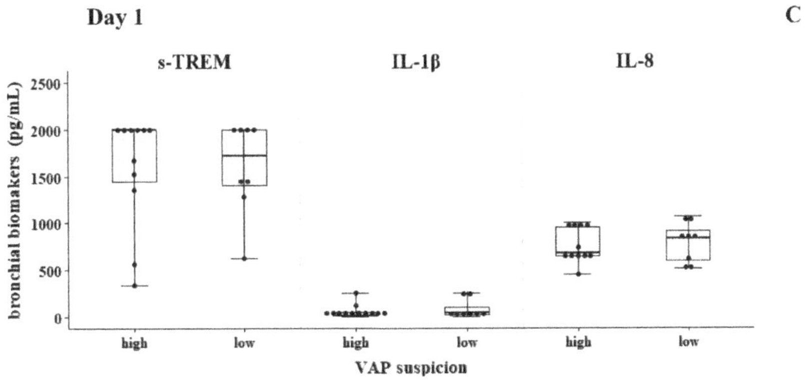

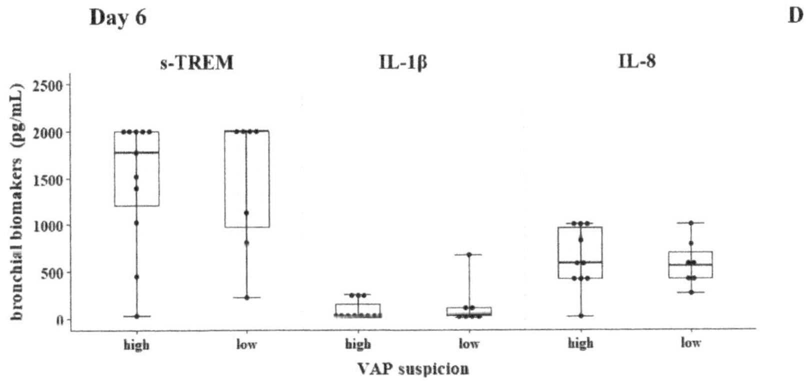

Figure 2. PTX-3, SP-D, s-TREM, IL-1β and IL-8 levels in bronchial aspirates of critically ill children with VAP suspicion. Concentrations of PTX-3 (ng/mL), SP-D (ng/mL), s-TREM (pg/mL), IL-1β (pg/mL) and IL-8 (pg/mL) in bronchial aspirates from patients with VAP suspicion on a mechanical ventilator at days 1 and 6 are shown (panels (**A–D**)). Statistically significant differences between the groups were examined using the non-parametric Kruskal-Wallis ANOVA test with Dunn's multiple comparisons test.

Correlation between blood and bronchial levels of biomarkers: At patient level, no significant correlation was found between blood and bronchial SP-D levels for patients with high VAP suspicion on day 1 (r = −0.133; p = 0.68) and on day 6 (r = 0.2; p = 0.555): Figure 3, panel A). In addition, for patients with low VAP suspicion also there was no correlation between the levels of blood and bronchial SP-D levels on day 1 (r = 0.37; p = 0.46) or day 6 (r = 0.51; p = 0.24): Figure 3, panel B. Similarly, no correlation was found between blood and bronchial PTX-3 levels in the high VAP suspicion group on day 1 (r = −0.048; p = 0.88) or day 6 (r = 0.42; p = 0.25): Figure 4, panel A. In the low VAP suspicion group r = 0.16 for day 1 (p = 0.69) and for day 6 r = −0.61 (p = 0.145): Figure 4, panel B.

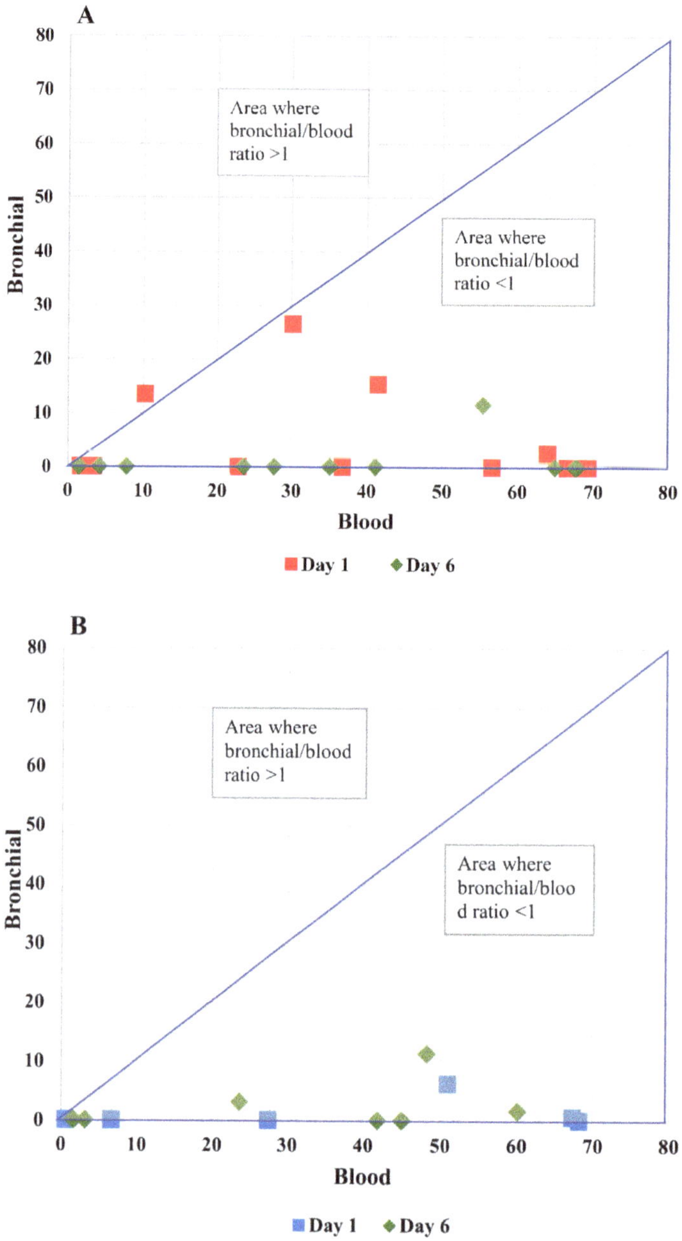

Figure 3. Bronchial vs. blood SP-D levels of critically ill children with high and low VAP suspicion. The SP-D level ratio between bronchial and blood samples on days 1 and 6 are shown for critically ill children with high (panel (**A**)) and low (panel (**B**)) VAP suspicion. The correlation coefficient between blood and bronchial SP-D levels (ng/mL) for patients with high VAP suspicion on day 1 (red square) was r = −0.133 (p = 0.68) and on day 6 (green diamond), r = 0.2 (p = 0.555). The correlation coefficient between blood and bronchial SP-D levels for patients with low VAP suspicion on day 1 (blue square) was r = 0.37 (p = 0.46) and on day 6 (green diamond), r = 0.51 (p = 0.24).

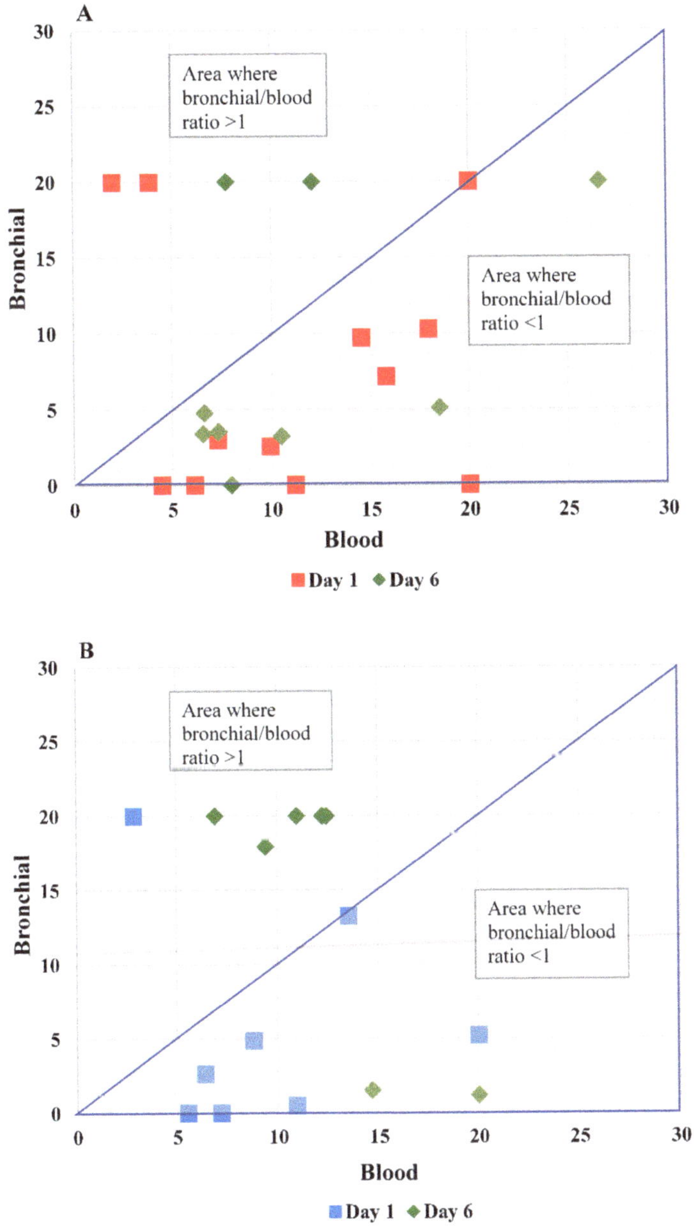

Figure 4. Bronchial vs. blood PTX-3 levels of critically ill children with high and low VAP suspicion. The PTX-3 level ratio between bronchial and blood samples in days 1 and 6 are shown for critically ill children with high (panel (**A**)) and low (panel (**B**)) VAP suspicion. The correlation coefficient between blood and bronchial PTX-3 levels (ng/mL) for patients with high VAP suspicion on day 1 (red square) was r = −0.048 (p = 0.88) and on day 6 (green diamond), r = 0.42 (p = 0.25). The correlation coefficient between blood and bronchial PTX-3 levels for patients with low VAP suspicion on day 1 (blue square) was r = 0.16 (p = 0.69) and on day 6 (green diamond), r = −0.61 (p = 0.145).

Correlation between the level of biomarkers and patient outcomes: Of all the biomarkers tested in this study (blood and bronchial), only the levels of IL-1β obtained on day 1 after enrollment correlated significantly with the number of mechanical ventilation days (r= 0.67; $p < 0.001$) and PICU stay (r = 0.66; $p < 0.002$).

Mortality was recorded for 2/20 patients only in the high VAP suspicion group ($p = 0.49$). One death happened 30 days after ICU discharge, whereas the other death occurred on day 3 of the study following a severe sepsis episode.

3. Discussion

In this prospective, pragmatic study conducted under real-life routine clinical practice conditions on mechanically ventilated critically ill children with suspicion of ventilator-associated pneumonia, biomarkers in the blood and bronchial aspirates of patients with a high or low suspicion of VAP diagnosis could not be discriminated. However, both the length of mechanical ventilation and ICU stay correlated significantly with the levels of IL-1β measured in bronchial aspirates on day 1 of VAP suspicion.

A gold standard for VAP diagnosis is still missing [6,19], and this has important implications for research into the epidemiology, natural history, treatment and prevention of VAP, especially in children. Although there is a shift toward more objective criteria in VAP diagnosis using the current ventilator-associated event (VAE) definitions, the new algorithm was developed mostly for epidemiological issues, not for clinical use [23]. Most research on VAP in children has been based on radiological definitions such as CDC pneumonia criteria and the CPIS [6]. A number of studies have shown the sensitivity and specificity of these definitions, including the mCPIS, for children [24–27]. In this study, children were enrolled with a different level of VAP suspicion, thereby avoiding the use of a specific definition that would bias our result and discriminate patients according to predefined criteria in the absence of a gold-standard definition.

As research into the implementation of fast-track diagnostics using syndromic panels grows, especially in ICU settings, it has been shown that molecular platforms have the potential to improve antimicrobial use and benefit patient outcomes compared to standard culture methods [28]. In our study, we used both bronchial aspirate cultures to identify and monitor detected bacteria as other studies have done, but we also employed rapid syndromic molecular diagnostics to identify potential pathogens such as viruses, non-culturable microorganisms and antimicrobial resistance profiles. Most of our patients had a negative molecular test, suggesting that VAP suspicion was clinically rather than microbiologically driven.

CRP is synthesized in the liver in response to the increased release of inflammatory cytokines at the site of the disease. Although its role in diagnostics includes a delay in responding to clinical stimuli and poor specificity—as increased CRP levels are found in a variety of pathologies other than VAP—studies have shown that it is a robust biomarker for acute-phase conditions [29]. In our study, two non-colonized patients of the low VAP suspicion group with declining CRP levels developed sepsis, increasing CRP levels at least threefold between the two monitored timepoints. Large clinical studies conducted with adult populations demonstrated its clinical value in hospital admissions because increased serum CRP levels have been significantly associated with increased 30-day mortality and need for mechanical ventilation [30], whereas monitoring CRP levels often seems to be useful for the early prediction of VAP [31]. However, the clinical value of CRP levels combined with PRISMIII to predict early VAP diagnosis in the pediatric population seems to be limited [32]. In our study, we also found no significant differences in the CRP serum levels measured at four timepoints between the high and low VAP groups. As the diagnostic accuracy may have been affected by the small sample size, the next step would be to enlarge the sample size and monitor CRP levels daily to evaluate the clinical utility of CRP in early VAP diagnosis.

This is the first time that PTX-3 levels had been evaluated simultaneously and repeatedly in both bronchial aspirates and serum in children with VAP suspicion. Tekerek et al. found that PTX-3 serum levels were significantly higher in pediatric patients with microbiologically confirmed VAP compared to children with suspected VAP and controls, where an optimal cut-off value for PTX-3 in serum was reported to be 4.19 ng/mL. The mCPIS was used for VAP diagnosis [13]. In our study, using the mCPIS score for patient classification, we found that the majority of patients with high and low suspicion of VAP had PTX-3 serum levels above the aforementioned cut-off value and the difference between the two groups was not significant. This could have been attributed to a different case mix but also to subjective limitations seen in mCPIS [33]. In addition, we found no correlation between the blood and bronchial levels of PTX-3 in patients with high or low VAP suspicion on day 1 or day 6. Two other studies conducted in adult patients with VAP found a cut-off value for PTX-3 in serum to be 16.43 and 2.56 ng/mL [34,35]. Only in one of these studies were serum PTX-3 levels measured sequentially starting from the day of intubation [34] In our pragmatic study, serial measurements of PTX-3 levels in serum remained elevated (6–10 ng/mL) among children with high and low suspicion of VAP probably because of other factors that may have influenced these levels.

The measurement of SP-D serum levels had been evaluated previously in one study and were proven to be the most sensitive biomarker for VAP diagnosis in critically ill children [13]. The cut-off value for this study was found to be 137.25 ng/mL, which was too high for our study population. All of our patients with either high or low VAP suspicion had a much lower SP-D level (6–42 ng/mL) during all four sequential serum measurements within the 12-day interval after VAP suspicion and study enrollment. Such value diversity calls for the validation of the optimal cut-off values for numerous serum biomarkers, including SP-D and PTX-3, in multicenter cohort studies of ventilated pediatric patients using a standard methodology.

The use of biomarkers in lower respiratory tract samples is attractive for most physicians and has been explored in many adult and a few pediatric studies [6,13,36,37]. In our study, five biomarkers—s-TREM, SP-D, PTX-3, IL-1β and IL-8—were for the first time simultaneously measured in bronchial aspirates of critically ill children with suspected VAP at two timepoints. Among these biomarkers, s-TREM was evaluated in four studies, three pediatric [20–22] and one neonatal [38], with conflicting results concerning the cut-off values of s-TREM for VAP diagnosis. Similarly, SP-D levels in BAL were evaluated in two pediatric studies [14,22] with conflicting conclusions regarding the clinical value of this biomarker. Specifically, one study concluded that SP-D has poor discriminatory power between VAP and colonization [22], whereas the second reported that elevated BAL SP-D levels represented a robust indication for a presumed nosocomial inoculation [14]. In addition, our study found no correlation between the levels of SP-D in bronchial aspirates and blood for either patient group. This indicated that using both bronchial and serum levels may not have helped to discriminate patients with or without VAP and that more data are needed to evaluate the role (if any) and the corresponding cut-off values of SP-D in children with VAP.

The inflammatory mediators IL-8 and IL-1β have been evaluated only in adult patients as part of a panel of biomarkers having the potential to correctly classify VAP cases from patients with brain injury or ventilated patients with non-pulmonary sepsis [39,40]. The authors concluded that patients who developed VAP had increased levels of these biomarkers, reflecting an inflammatory response to infection without however being able to differentiate VAP pneumonia in patients with brain injury or non-pulmonary sepsis. Nevertheless, a prospective multicenter study in 12 adult ICUs showed that low concentrations of IL-1β and IL-8 in BAL samples can confidently exclude VAP [36]. In our study, although none of these biomarkers had a predictive role for VAP diagnosis, IL-1β levels on day 1 were associated with mechanical ventilation and ICU stay. The use of endpoint clinical characteristics such as morbidity and mortality may have a more predictive, prognostic role as well as an added value for the patient besides exploring the validity of a current or new VAP algorithm [23,41]. Combining existing VAP diagnostic modules (including biomarkers) and exploring the best association with patient outcomes may be the best way to identify potential modifiable factors that would improve quality improvement in ventilated critically ill children [23]. However, this needs to be supported by multi-center and large-scale studies in children.

The strengths include rigorous inclusion criteria, collection of detailed information on standard of care testing and clinical outcomes as well as detailed assessment of both microbiological and molecular specimen testing for patient enrollment. The limitations of this study are the small number of patients and the antibiotic administration to all patients during the study enrollment. The latter could have led to borderline cases that influenced the overall expression levels of biomarkers in bronchial aspirates or blood. The fact that the bronchial/blood ratios were found to be non-discriminatory could have been due to the unequal compartmentalization of PTX-3 and SP-D at the time of sample collection. Although the children in this study were classified on the basis of VAP suspicion using the mCPIS score, the subjectivity and sensitivity of the score has been criticized [33]. However, it has been used in most studies exploring VAP diagnosis both in children and adults as well as in clinical practice [6]. The potentially missing of culture-based identified VAP pathogens was minimized by implementing multiplex PCR-based syndromic panel diagnostics. In addition, viral VAP, although rare, has clinical features that cannot be easily differentiated from bacterial infection [42].

In conclusion, the results of this study, supported by the existing literature, so far show that the clinical value of using biomarkers to diagnose VAP in critically ill children remains suggestive. The implementation of molecular diagnostics using syndromic panels to detect VAP-associated pathogens, especially in ICU settings, seems to benefit patient outcomes compared to standard culture methods. There is an urgent need for large multicenter cohort studies to set the baseline levels of candidate biomarkers to minimize selection bias and focus on outcomes such as morbidity and mortality.

4. Materials and Methods

Study design and Patient population: This was a single-center prospective pilot cohort study conducted from March 2021 to December 2022 on mechanically ventilated critically ill children in an 8-bed multivalent PICU of a tertiary university-affiliated hospital. Children between 1 month and 14 years of age with clinical suspicion of VAP and on mechanical ventilation for at least 48 h were eligible for enrollment, after their parents or guardians signed an informed consent form. To reflect an typical real-life scenario in pediatric critical care, enrollment was based on three tailor-made ICU criteria for VAP suspicion: (1) purulent respiratory or positive bronchial aspirate culture and the initiation of antimicrobial agent(s) for suspicion of VAP infection according to local practice; (2) increased oxygen requirement (defined as >20%) and fever, hypothermia, leukocytosis or leukopenia, and the initiation of antimicrobial agent(s); and (3) radiological findings of new lung infiltrates and at least 2 criteria from the following: fever (>38 °C) or hypothermia (<36 °C), increase in oxygen requirement >20%, purulent respiratory secretions, white blood cells count <4 or $>12 \times 10^9$ cells/L and CRP > 10 mg/L. Patients were excluded if (1) informed consent was declined, (2) the patient was unlikely to survive 48 h after enrollment, (3) pregnancy had occurred for adolescent female subjects, and (4) if body weight was less than 3 kg. On day 1 of the study for all enrolled patients, the modified CPIS (mCPIS) tool for VAP diagnosis was used [33] to assign them to one of two groups: a high VAP suspicion (mCPIS > 6) and a low VAP suspicion (mCPIS < 6).

Data and sample collection: Patient data recorded on standard electronic case report forms included demographic, clinical, chest radiograph and culture data. PRISMIII scoring was used for mortality risk assessment and the mCPIS score for VAP diagnosis and management (Table 1). Blood samples for hematological and biochemical measurements were collected at 4 time points corresponding to days 1, 3, 6 and 12 after the onset of event. Bronchial samples collected by expert PICU practitioners were liquefied in a sterile 0.9% saline solution and divided into three aliquots: two were processed immediately for microbiological and molecular diagnostics analysis, and the other was frozen at −75 °C for biomarker assay measurements. Bronchial aliquots were cultured 30 min after collection.

Culture procedures: The collected samples were inoculated on blood and MacConkey agar by using sterile inoculating loop. After incubation at 37 °C for 24–48 h, bacterial growth was measured and colony counts $\geq 10^4$ CFU/mL were considered as the diagnostic threshold for infection. Species identification and susceptibility testing were determined by conventional means using the VITEK-2 automated system (bioMérieux, Marcy l' Étoile, France).

Molecular diagnostics analysis: For rapid molecular diagnostics, bronchial aliquots were analyzed using the Biofire Filmarray pneumonia plus panel (bioMérieux) run on a multiplexed PCR-based diagnostic platform to test for the presence of 27 of the most common pathogens involved in lower respiratory tract infections and to identify antibiotic resistance markers: $bla_{CTX\text{-}M}$, bla_{KPC}, bla_{NDM}, bla_{VIM}, $bla_{OXA48\text{-like}}$ and *Mec*A/*Mec*C genes. The cutoff value for colonization or infection was set at 10^4 copies/mL.

Biomarker analysis: Serum and bronchial samples obtained at the four time points were frozen at −75 °C until processed by a sandwich ELISA assay following the manufacturer's recommendations (Proteintech Group, Manchester, UK). The samples were diluted (four-fold for PTX-3 detection and two-fold for s-TREM, IL-1β and IL-8 measurements) and run in duplicate on a 96-well format. Final protein concentrations were obtained by being multiplied by the respective dilution factors. The range of detection for each protein tested was: 0.027–20 ng/mL for PTX-3, 31.25–2000 pg/mL for s-TREM, 3.9–250 pg/mL for IL-1 β and 15.6–1000 pg/mL for IL-8. The highest and lowest limits of each protein standard were used as sample values for the samples read as outliers by the assay. Protein concentrations for each biomarker and experimental condition were obtained using a four-parameter logistic regression curve fit.

Statistical analysis: Continuous variables were presented as mean ± SD and comparisons between the groups were determined using an unpaired Student's *t* or a Mann–Whitney U test depending on data distribution. Categorical values were expressed as percentages and comparisons were made using chi square or Fisher's exact tests.

A Spearman's correlation coefficient was used for correlation (a) between the levels of two biomarkers (PTX-3 and SPD) in blood and bronchial aspirates in patient for both high- and low-risk VAP groups for the same day, and (b) between the level of biomarkers (in blood or bronchial aspirates) and patient outcomes (length of mechanical ventilation, length of ICU stay, length of hospital stay, ICU and hospital mortality).

All data analysis was performed using the statistics program Instat (GraphPad, Inc., San Diego, CA, USA) and IBM SPSS v28 software package. A two-tailed p value < 0.05 was considered statistically significant.

Author Contributions: M.S. (Maria Sdougka), E.V. and A.V. were involved in sample and medical record data collection. V.G. was involved in the examination, evaluation and interpretation of radiographic data. A.F. was involved in data curation. M.S. (Maria Simitsopoulou) was involved in experimental design and result acquisition, statistical analysis, writing original draft of the manuscript, final editing and formatting. E.R. was involved in proofreading. E.I. was involved in funding acquisition, project administration, supervision, statistical analysis, final editing and formatting of the manuscript. All authors have read and agreed to the published version of the manuscript.

Funding: This research project was supported by the Hellenic Foundation for Research and Innovation (H.F.R.I.) under the "2nd Call for H.F.R.I. Research Projects to support Post-Doctoral Researchers" (Project Number: 1047).

Institutional Review Board Statement: The study was conducted according to the guidelines of the Declaration of Helsinki and approved by the Ethics Committee of Hippokration General Hospital of Thessaloniki, protocol code: 58291/7.12.2020, date of approval: 14 April 2021.

Informed Consent Statement: Informed consent was obtained from all subjects enrolled in the study.

Data Availability Statement: We confirm that the data supporting the findings of this study are available on reasonable request.

Acknowledgments: The authors extend their appreciation to all PICU staff as well as to Maria Kitsou and Zoe Kravari for their overall assistance in this study.

Conflicts of Interest: Emmanuel Roilides reports fees to his institution from Amplyx, Astellas, Gilead, MSD, Pfizer, Scynexis, GSK and Shionogi, outside the submitted work. The remaining authors declare no conflict of interest.

References

1. Zingg, W.; Hopkins, S.; Gayet-Ageron, A.; Holmes, A.; Sharland, M.; Suetens, C.; group EP study. Health-care-associated infections in neonates, children, and adolescents: An analysis of paediatric data from the European Centre for Disease Prevention and Control point-prevalence survey. *Lancet Infect. Dis.* **2017**, *17*, 381–389. [CrossRef]
2. Gupta, S.; Boville, B.M.; Blanton, R.; Lukasiewicz, G.; Wincek, J.; Bai, C.; Forbes, M.L. A multicentered prospective analysis of diagnosis, risk factors, and outcomes associated with pediatric ventilator-associated pneumonia. *Pediatr. Crit. Care Med.* **2015**, *16*, e65–e73. [CrossRef] [PubMed]
3. Melsen, W.G.; Rovers, M.M.; Groenwold, R.H.; Bergmans, D.C.; Camus, C.; Bauer, T.T.; Hanisch, E.W.; Klarin, B.; Koeman, M.; Krueger, W.A.; et al. Attributable mortality of ventilator-associated pneumonia: A meta-analysis of individual patient data from randomised prevention studies. *Lancet Infect. Dis.* **2013**, *13*, 665–671. [CrossRef] [PubMed]
4. Hernandez-Garcia, M.; Girona-Alarcon, M.; Bobillo-Perez, S.; Urrea-Ayala, M.; Sole-Ribalta, A.; Balaguer, M.; Cambra, F.J.; Jordan, I. Ventilator-associated pneumonia is linked to a worse prognosis than community-acquired pneumonia in children. *PLoS ONE* **2022**, *17*, e0271450. [CrossRef] [PubMed]
5. Antalova, N.; Klucka, J.; Rihova, M.; Polackova, S.; Pokorna, A.; Stourac, P. Ventilator-Associated Pneumonia Prevention in Pediatric Patients: Narrative Review. *Children* **2022**, *9*, 1540. [CrossRef] [PubMed]
6. Iosifidis, E.; Pitsava, G.; Roilides, E. Ventilator-associated pneumonia in neonates and children: A systematic analysis of diagnostic methods and prevention. *Future Microbiol.* **2018**, *13*, 1431–1446. [CrossRef]
7. Network NNHS. Pneumonia (Ventilator-Associated [VAP] and Non-Ventilator-Associated Pneumonia [PNEU]) Event. 2023. 1–19. Available online: https://www.cdc.gov/nhsn/index.html (accessed on 24 March 2023).
8. van Wyk, L.; Applegate, J.T.; Salie, S. Ventilator-associated pneumonia in PICU-how are we doing? *S. Afr. J. Crit. Care* **2022**, *38*, 71–74. [CrossRef]
9. Venkatachalam, V.; Hendley, J.O.; Willson, D.F. The diagnostic dilemma of ventilator-associated pneumonia in critically ill children. *Pediatr. Crit. Care Med.* **2011**, *12*, 286–296. [CrossRef]
10. Coelho, L.; Rabello, L.; Salluh, J.; Martin-Loeches, I.; Rodriguez, A.; Nseir, S.; Gomes, J.A.; Povoa, P.; Group TAv study. C-reactive protein and procalcitonin profile in ventilator-associated lower respiratory infections. *J. Crit. Care* **2018**, *48*, 385–389. [CrossRef]
11. Luyt, C.E.; Combes, A.; Reynaud, C.; Hekimian, G.; Nieszkowska, A.; Tonnellier, M.; Aubry, A.; Trouillet, J.L.; Bernard, M.; Chastre, J. Usefulness of procalcitonin for the diagnosis of ventilator-associated pneumonia. *Intensive Care Med.* **2008**, *34*, 1434–1440. [CrossRef] [PubMed]
12. Palazzo, S.J.; Simpson, T.; Schnapp, L. Biomarkers for ventilator-associated pneumonia: Review of the literature. *Heart Lung* **2011**, *40*, 293–298. [CrossRef]
13. Tekerek, N.U.; Akyildiz, B.N.; Ercal, B.D.; Muhtaroglu, S. New Biomarkers to Diagnose Ventilator Associated Pneumonia: Pentraxin 3 and Surfactant Protein D. *Indian J. Pediatr.* **2018**, *85*, 426–432. [CrossRef] [PubMed]
14. Said, A.S.; Abd-Elaziz, M.M.; Farid, M.M.; Abd-ElFattah, M.A.; Abdel-Monim, M.T.; Doctor, A. Evolution of surfactant protein-D levels in children with ventilator-associated pneumonia. *Pediatr. Pulmonol.* **2012**, *47*, 292–299. [CrossRef] [PubMed]
15. Refaat, A.; Affara, N.; Abdel-fatah, W.; Hussein, T.; El-gerbi, M. Diagnostic accuracy of inflammatory biomarkers in bronchoalveolar lavage from patients with ventilator-associated pneumonia. *Egypt. J. Chest Dis. Tuberc.* **2014**, *63*, 723–730. [CrossRef]
16. Fagon, J.Y. Biological markers and diagnosis of ventilator-associated pneumonia. *Crit. Care* **2011**, *15*, 130. [CrossRef] [PubMed]
17. Salluh, J.I.F.; Souza-Dantas, V.C.; Povoa, P. The current status of biomarkers for the diagnosis of nosocomial pneumonias. *Curr. Opin. Crit. Care* **2017**, *23*, 391–397. [CrossRef] [PubMed]
18. Ratageri, V.H.; Panigatti, P.; Mukherjee, A.; Das, R.R.; Goyal, J.P.; Bhat, J.I.; Vyas, B.; Lodha, R.; Singhal, D.; Kumar, P.; et al. Role of procalcitonin in diagnosis of community acquired pneumonia in Children. *BMC Pediatr.* **2022**, *22*, 217. [CrossRef]
19. Kalil, A.C.; Metersky, M.L.; Klompas, M.; Muscedere, J.; Sweeney, D.A.; Palmer, L.B.; Napolitano, L.M.; O'Grady, N.P.; Bartlett, J.G.; Carratala, J.; et al. Management of Adults With Hospital-acquired and Ventilator-associated Pneumonia: 2016 Clinical Practice Guidelines by the Infectious Diseases Society of America and the American Thoracic Society. *Clin. Infect. Dis.* **2016**, *63*, e61–e111. [CrossRef]
20. Isguder, R.; Ceylan, G.; Agin, H.; Gulfidan, G.; Ayhan, Y.; Devrim, I. New parameters for childhood ventilator associated pneumonia diagnosis. *Pediatr. Pulmonol.* **2017**, *52*, 119–128. [CrossRef] [PubMed]
21. Matsuno, A.K.; Carlotti, A.P. Role of soluble triggering receptor expressed on myeloid cells-1 for diagnosing ventilator-associated pneumonia after cardiac surgery: An observational study. *BMC Cardiovasc. Disord.* **2013**, *13*, 107. [CrossRef]
22. Srinivasan, R.; Song, Y.; Wiener-Kronish, J.; Flori, H.R. Plasminogen activation inhibitor concentrations in bronchoalveolar lavage fluid distinguishes ventilator-associated pneumonia from colonization in mechanically ventilated pediatric patients. *Pediatr. Crit. Care Med.* **2011**, *12*, 21–27. [CrossRef] [PubMed]

23. Iosifidis, E.; Coffin, S. Ventilator-associated Events in Children: Controversies and Research Needs. *Pediatr. Infect. Dis. J.* **2020**, *39*, e37–e39. [CrossRef] [PubMed]
24. Larsson, J.; Itenov, T.S.; Bestle, M.H. Risk prediction models for mortality in patients with ventilator-associated pneumonia: A systematic review and meta-analysis. *J. Crit. Care* **2017**, *37*, 112–118. [CrossRef] [PubMed]
25. Pelosi, P.; Barassi, A.; Severgnini, P.; Gomiero, B.; Finazzi, S.; Merlini, G.; d'Eril, G.M.; Chiaranda, M.; Niederman, M.S. Prognostic role of clinical and laboratory criteria to identify early ventilator-associated pneumonia in brain injury. *Chest* **2008**, *134*, 101–108. [CrossRef]
26. Schurink, C.A.M.; Nieuwenhoven, C.A.V.; Jacobs, J.A.; Rozenberg-Arska, M.; Joore, H.C.A.; Buskens, E.; Hoepelman, A.I.M.; Bonten, M.J.M. Clinical pulmonary infection score for ventilator-associated pneumonia: Accuracy and inter-observer variability. *Intensive Care Med.* **2004**, *30*, 217–224. [CrossRef]
27. Zilberberg, M.D.; Shorr, A.F. Ventilator-associated pneumonia: The clinical pulmonary infection score as a surrogate for diagnostics and outcome. *Clin. Infect. Dis.* **2010**, *1* (Suppl. 51), S131–S135. [CrossRef]
28. Calderaro, A.; Buttrini, M.; Farina, B.; Montecchini, S.; De Conto, F.; Chezzi, C. Respiratory Tract Infections and Laboratory Diagnostic Methods: A Review with A Focus on Syndromic Panel-Based Assays. *Microorganisms* **2022**, *10*, 1856. [CrossRef]
29. Karakioulaki, M.; Stolz, D. Biomarkers in Pneumonia-Beyond Procalcitonin. *Int. J. Mol. Sci.* **2019**, *20*, 2004. [CrossRef]
30. Chalmers, J.D.; Singanayagam, A.; Hill, A.T. C-reactive protein is an independent predictor of severity in community-acquired pneumonia. *Am. J. Med.* **2008**, *121*, 219–225. [CrossRef]
31. Povoa, P.; Martin-Loeches, I.; Ramirez, P.; Bos, L.D.; Esperatti, M.; Silvestre, J.; Gili, G.; Goma, G.; Berlanga, E.; Espasa, M.; et al. Biomarker kinetics in the prediction of VAP diagnosis: Results from the BioVAP study. *Ann. Intensive Care* **2016**, *6*, 32. [CrossRef]
32. Sun, Y.; Zhao, T.; Li, D.; Huo, J.; Hu, L.; Xu, F. Predictive value of C-reactive protein and the Pediatric Risk of Mortality III Score for occurrence of postoperative ventilator-associated pneumonia in pediatric patients with congenital heart disease. *Pediatr. Investig.* **2019**, *3*, 91–95. [CrossRef]
33. da Silva, P.S.; de Aguiar, V.E.; de Carvalho, W.B.; Machado Fonseca, M.C. Value of clinical pulmonary infection score in critically ill children as a surrogate for diagnosis of ventilator-associated pneumonia. *J. Crit. Care* **2014**, *29*, 545–550. [CrossRef] [PubMed]
34. Bilgin, H.; Haliloglu, M.; Yaman, A.; Ay, P.; Bilgili, B.; Arslantas, M.K.; Ture Ozdemir, F.; Haklar, G.; Cinel, I.; Mulazimoglu, L. Sequential Measurements of Pentraxin 3 Serum Levels in Patients with Ventilator-Associated Pneumonia: A Nested Case-Control Study. *Can. J. Infect. Dis. Med. Microbiol.* **2018**, *2018*, 4074169. [CrossRef]
35. Lin, Q.; Fu, F.; Shen, L.; Zhu, B. Pentraxin 3 in the assessment of ventilator-associated pneumonia: An early marker of severity. *Heart Lung* **2013**, *42*, 139–145. [CrossRef] [PubMed]
36. Hellyer, T.P.; Morris, A.C.; McAuley, D.F.; Walsh, T.S.; Anderson, N.H.; Singh, S.; Dark, P.; Roy, A.I.; Baudouin, S.V.; Wright, S.E.; et al. Diagnostic accuracy of pulmonary host inflammatory mediators in the exclusion of ventilator-acquired pneumonia. *Thorax* **2015**, *70*, 41–47. [CrossRef]
37. Ye, W.; Huang, Q.D.; Tang, T.Y.; Qin, G.Y. Diagnostic value of pentraxin 3 in respiratory tract infections: A meta-analysis. *Medicine* **2020**, *99*, e19532. [CrossRef]
38. Zhao, X.; Xu, L.; Yang, Z.; Sun, B.; Wang, Y.; Li, G.; Feng, C.; Pan, T.; Yu, T.; Feng, X. Significance of sTREM-1 in early prediction of ventilator-associated pneumonia in neonates: A single-center, prospective, observational study. *BMC Infect. Dis.* **2020**, *20*, 542. [CrossRef] [PubMed]
39. Antcliffe, D.B.; Wolfer, A.M.; O'Dea, K.P.; Takata, M.; Holmes, E.; Gordon, A.C. Profiling inflammatory markers in patients with pneumonia on intensive care. *Sci. Rep.* **2018**, *8*, 14736. [CrossRef]
40. Grover, V.; Pantelidis, P.; Soni, N.; Takata, M.; Shah, P.L.; Wells, A.U.; Henderson, D.C.; Kelleher, P.; Singh, S. A biomarker panel (Bioscore) incorporating monocytic surface and soluble TREM-1 has high discriminative value for ventilator-associated pneumonia: A prospective observational study. *PLoS ONE* **2014**, *9*, e109686. [CrossRef]
41. Rello, J.; Bunsow, E. What is the Research Agenda in Ventilator-associated Pneumonia? *Int. J. Infect. Dis.* **2016**, *51*, 110–112. [CrossRef]
42. Shorr, A.F.; Ilges, D.T.; Micek, S.T.; Kollef, M.H. The importance of viruses in ventilator-associated pneumonia. *Infect. Control Hosp. Epidemiol.* 2022; 1–6, *online ahead of print*.

antibiotics

MDPI

Article

Replacement of the Double Meropenem Disc Test with a Lateral Flow Assay for the Detection of Carbapenemase-Producing Enterobacterales and *Pseudomonas aeruginosa* in Clinical Laboratory Practice

Areti Tychala, Georgios Meletis *, Paraskevi Mantzana, Angeliki Kassomenaki, Charikleia Katsanou, Aikaterini Daviti, Lydia Kouroudi, Lemonia Skoura and Efthymia Protonotariou

Department of Microbiology, AHEPA University Hospital, School of Medicine, Aristotle University of Thessaloniki, S. Kiriakidi Str. 1, 54636 Thessaloniki, Greece; aretich@gmail.com (A.T.)
* Correspondence: meletisg@hotmail.com; Tel.: +30-6974282575

Abstract: The prompt detection of carbapenemases among Gram-negative bacteria isolated from patients' clinical infection samples and surveillance cultures is important for the implementation of infection control measures. In this context, we evaluated the effectiveness of replacing phenotypic tests for the detection of carbapenemase producers with the immunochromatographic Carbapenem-Resistant K.N.I.V.O. Detection K-Set lateral flow assay (LFA). In total, 178 carbapenem-resistant Enterobacterales and 32 carbapenem-resistant *Pseudomonas aeruginosa* isolated in our hospital were tested with both our established phenotypic and molecular testing procedures and the LFA. The Kappa coefficient of agreement for Enterobacterales was 0.85 ($p < 0.001$) and 0.6 ($p < 0.001$) for *P. aeruginosa*. No major disagreements were observed and notably, in many cases, the LFA detected more carbapenemases than the double meropenem disc test, especially regarding OXA-48 in Enterobacterales and VIM in *P. aeruginosa*. Overall, the Carbapenem-Resistant K.N.I.V.O. Detection K-Set was very effective and at least equivalent to the standard procedures used in our lab. However, it was much faster as it provided results in 15 min compared to a minimum of 18–24 h for the phenotypic tests.

Keywords: *Klebsiella pneumoniae*; *Pseudomonas aeruginosa*; carbapenemases; NDM; KPC; IMP; VIM; OXA-48; LFA

1. Introduction

β-lactam antibiotics are widely used in medical practice because of their effectiveness and their limited adverse effects [1]. They share a common β-lactam ring and act by binding to and inactivating the penicillin-binding proteins (PBPs), thus inhibiting bacterial cell wall formation. This category includes penicillins, cephalosporins, monobactams, and carbapenems, which are the most effective among the β-lactams and are less susceptible to the mechanisms of acquired bacterial resistance [2]. Therefore, the emergence and spread of carbapenem resistance is considered of major importance for public health [3]. Even though carbapenem resistance may be multi-factorial [4], the major resistance determinant against carbapenems among Gram-negative nosocomial pathogens is the production of enzymes able to hydrolyze these agents together with other β-lactams. These enzymes are commonly encoded by genes that are harbored in mobile genetic elements capable of horizontal gene transfer and consequent rapid dissemination [5].

Generally, all enzymes with the potential to hydrolyze at least some β-lactam antibiotics are called β-lactamases [6]. β-lactamases are categorized into four distinct molecular classes according to the Ambler classification [7]; class A, C, and D enzymes have serine in their active center, whereas class B have zinc in their active center and are, therefore, called metallo-beta-lactamases (MBLs). Enzymes of all classes that are able to hydrolyze carbapenems together with other β-lactam antibiotics are called carbapenemases [8,9]. Among class A enzymes, *Klebsiella pneumoniae* carbapenemases (KPCs) [10,11] are the most clinically important and have spread worldwide. Similarly, among class D representatives, oxacillinase-48 (OXA-48) and OXA-48-like enzymes have a wide global distribution [12]. Class B [13] includes, among other carbapenemases, imipenemases (IMPs) [14], Verona integron-encoded metallo-β-lactamases (VIMs) [15], and New Delhi metallo-β-lactamases (NDMs) [16]. Class C enzymes are not considered carbapenemases; some of them, however, may present a low potential of carbapenem hydrolysis and their overproduction may contribute to carbapenem resistance combined with diminished outer membrane permeability and/or efflux pump over-expression [17]. Overall, the most effective carbapenemases, in terms of carbapenem hydrolysis and geographical spread, are KPC, VIM, IMP, NDM, and OXA-48 types [18].

KPCs present with some specific characteristics. They inactivate all β-lactam antibiotics, are only partially inhibited by older β-lactamase inhibitors, such as clavulanic acid, tazobactam, and boronic acid, and are commonly inhibited by novel inhibitors, such as avibactam, relebactam, and vaborbactam. In phenotypic tests they are inhibited by phenylboronic acid but not ethylene diamine tetraacetic acid (EDTA). MBLs, on the other hand, can hydrolyze all β-lactams except aztreonam and cefiderocol, whereas they are not inhibited by the aforementioned β-lactamase inhibitors or by phenylboronic acid. Since they bear zinc in their active center, their in vitro inhibition is achieved by metal chelators, such as EDTA. Among them, NDM-type enzymes present unique features. They hydrolyze aztreonam and they commonly present negative modified Hodge test results [19].

The rapid and accurate identification of carbapenemase production among Gram-negative isolates recovered by patient infections or surveillance cultures is important for both therapeutic and infection control purposes. Several culture and non-culture based diagnostic tests have been developed. Non-culture methods include the molecular detection of carbapenemase-related genes, the biochemical detection of carbapenem hydrolysis, and antibody-based methods such as lateral flow immunoassays (LFA) for carbapenemase identification. Molecular assays such as multiple polymerase chain reaction (PCR) and loop-mediated isothermal amplification (LAMP) can rapidly detect and discriminate between different types of carbapenemase genes. Nevertheless, such methods require special equipment and are expensive. On the contrary, a lateral flow immunoassay (LFA) is a simple, rapid, and relatively low-cost method that could be used instead of the above expensive examples. Recently, several lateral flow assays have been introduced worldwide for the rapid and easy detection of multiple carbapenemases, substantially reducing the turnaround time compared to conventional culture-based methods [20].

Therefore, we evaluated the effectiveness of replacing phenotypic assays for the detection of carbapenemase producers with the new Carbapenem-Resistant K.N.I.V.O. Detection K-Set multiplex lateral flow assay developed by Goldstream, Beijing Gold Mountain river Tech Development Co., Ltd. (Beijing, China). For this purpose, we tested carbapenem resistant Enterobacterales and *Pseudomonas aeruginosa* isolated in our hospital with both our established phenotypic and molecular testing procedures and the LFA.

2. Results

In total, 210 single patient isolates were tested using both the double meropenem disc test (DMDT) and the K.N.I.V.O. Detection K-Set LFA. Among the studied isolates, 178 were Enterobacterales (155 *K. pneumoniae*, 10 *Proteus mirabilis*, 9 *Providencia stuartii*, 2 *Escherichia coli*, 1 *Klebsiella oxytoca*, and 1 *Enterobacter cloacae* complex) and 32 were *Pseudomonas aeruginosa*. The Enterobacterales were isolated from blood cultures (n = 67), urine samples (n = 40), bronchoalveolar secretions (n = 30), wound samples (n = 6), central venous catheters (n = 9), pleural fluid (n = 1), pus samples (n = 1), and rectal swabs (n = 24) taken for surveillance purposes at patient admission or during hospitalization. *P. aeruginosa* isolates were recovered from 18 blood cultures (n = 18), 5 urine samples (n = 5), bronchoalveolar secretions (n = 3), soft tissue infections (n = 1), 2 central venous catheters (n = 2), pleural fluid (n = 1), pus samples (n = 1), and rectal swabs (n = 1). KPC, OXA-48, and MBL including VIM and NDM were detected among the Enterobacterales as shown in Supplementary Table S1 and Figures 1–4. The Kappa coefficient of agreement between the two methods was 0.85 ($p < 0.001$).

P. aeruginosa isolates were found to produce only the VIM carbapenemase (Supplementary Table S2 and Figure 5). The Kappa coefficient of agreement between the two methods for *P. aeruginosa* was 0.6 ($p < 0.001$).

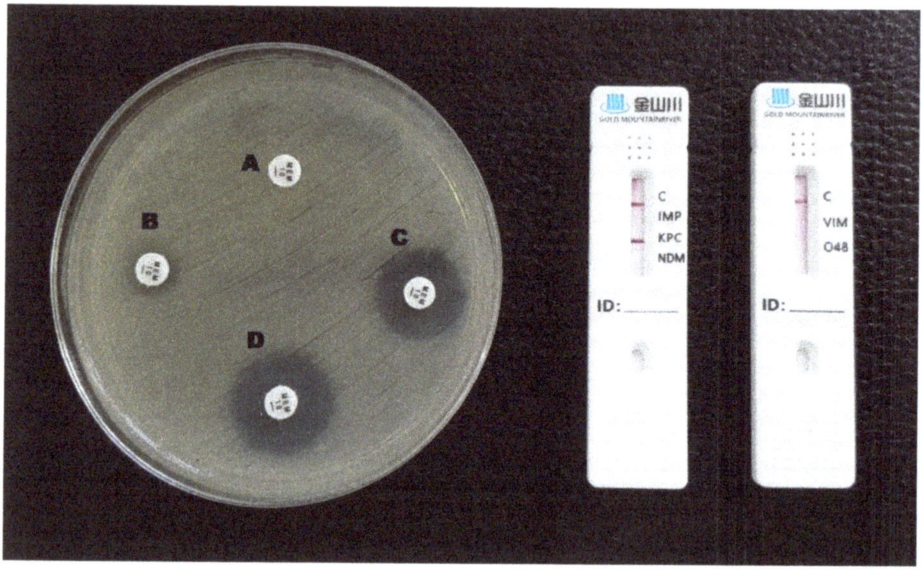

Figure 1. Phenotypic and lateral flow assay results for a KPC-producing *K. pneumoniae*. A: meropenem disc without inhibitors; B: meropenem + EDTA; C: meropenem + phenylboronic acid; D: meropenem + EDTA + phenylboronic acid. A red line in the KPC test area is visible in the LFA.

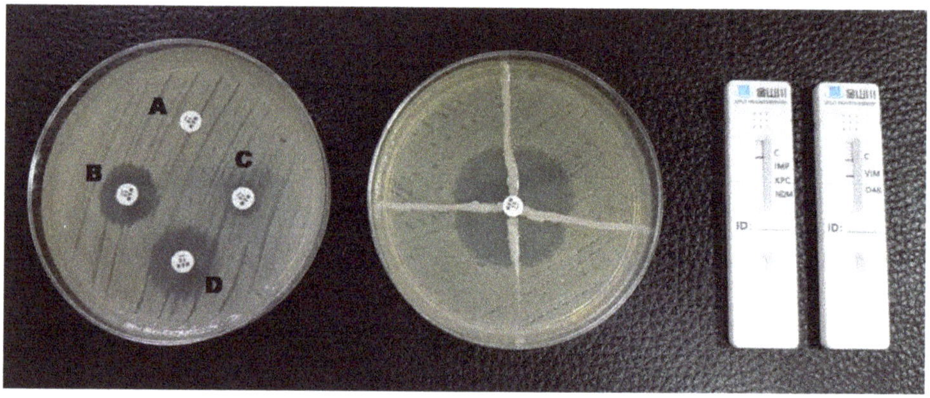

Figure 2. Phenotypic and lateral flow assay results for a VIM-producing *K. pneumoniae*. A: meropenem disc without inhibitors; B: meropenem + EDTA; C: meropenem + phenylboronic acid; D: meropenem + EDTA + phenylboronic acid. The Hodge test was positive and a red line in the VIM test area is visible in the LFA.

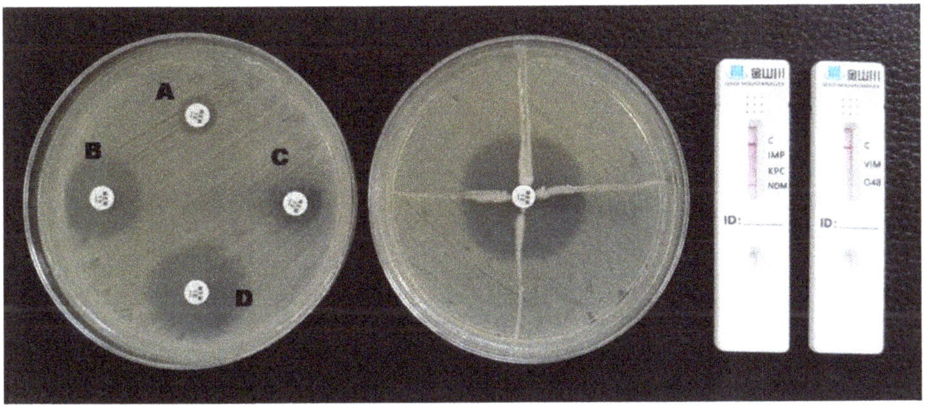

Figure 3. Phenotypic and lateral flow assay results for an NDM-producing *K. pneumoniae*. A: meropenem disc without inhibitors; B: meropenem + EDTA; C: meropenem + phenylboronic acid; D: meropenem + EDTA + phenylboronic acid. The Hodge test was negative and a red line in the NDM test area is visible in the LFA.

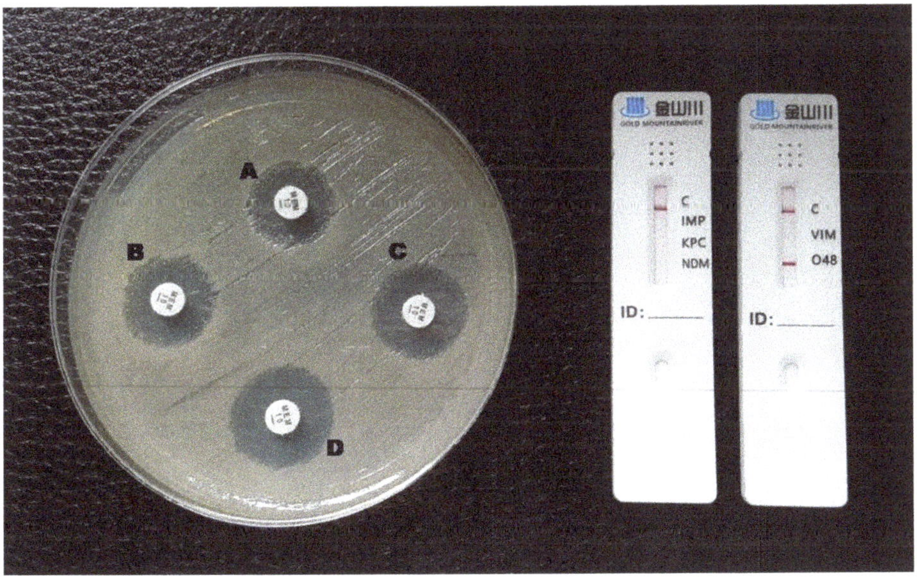

Figure 4. Phenotypic and lateral flow assay results for an OXA-48-producing *K. pneumoniae*. A: meropenem disc without inhibitors; B: meropenem + EDTA; C: meropenem + phenylboronic acid; D: meropenem + EDTA + phenylboronic acid. The test could not be interpreted by the double meropenem disc test (indeterminate) and a red line in the O48 test area is visible in the LFA.

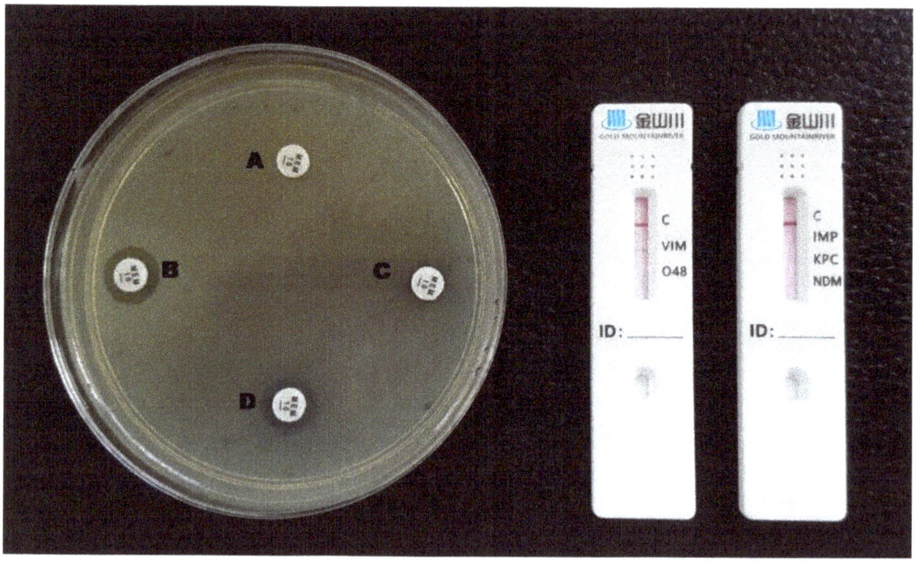

Figure 5. Phenotypic and lateral flow assay results for a VIM-producing *P. aeruginosa*. A: meropenem disc without inhibitors; B: meropenem + EDTA; C: meropenem + phenylboronic acid; D: meropenem + EDTA + phenylboronic acid. A red line in the VIM test area is visible in the LFA.

3. Discussion

In recent years, rapid diagnostic testing using LFAs for the detection of enzymes associated with antimicrobial resistance have been widely developed as they demonstrate comparable performance with gold standard PCR-based methods and can be easily applied in clinical microbiology laboratories without requiring specialized personnel and excessive cost [21–25].

In our study, the performance of K.N.V.I.O. for Enterobacterales was very good since the Kappa coefficient for Enterobacterales showed a strong agreement between the two methods. In fact, the level of agreement could have been even better; however, the presence of OXA-48 carbapenemases that were detected by the LFA and not detected by the DMDT biased the Kappa coefficient result. Indeed, the presence of OXA-48 cannot be detected by the DMDT; thus, the respective result is commonly indeterminate and cannot be interpreted. Of interest, there were no major disagreements between the two methods (for KPC instead of MBL) that could imply failures in the performance of the LFA. Moreover, in many cases, the LFA detected more carbapenemases than the DMDT could have done.

The Kappa coefficient for *P. aeruginosa* showed moderate agreement and this is exclusively because of the limitations of the DMDT to accurately detect carbapenemases in this species. Carbapenem resistance in *P. aeruginosa* might be more influenced than in other clinically important species by additional mechanisms such as efflux pumps over-expression or porin loss [26]. This may explain the inability of the DMDT to detect the presence of carbapenemases, because the interpretation of the test is based on comparing the inhibition halo of meropenem with and without the presence of specific inhibitors, especially if the carbapenemase is expressed at low levels. On the other hand, LFAs do not present the same limitation, and this can explain the detection of the VIM carbapenemase in isolates where the DMDT was not able to detect them.

Overall, in our study the performance of the LFA was satisfactory and improved the turnaround times of our laboratory. First, the use of the LFA allowed for the immediate distinction between VIM and NDM metallo-β-lactamases without the need to perform the Hodge test and PCR. Specifically, the use of the Hodge test is often problematic because it frequently produces an uncertain interpretation and can be biased by the presence of additional carbapenemases. Second, the LFA, in some cases, detected more carbapenemases than the DMDT in Enterobacterales, including OXA-48. Specifically, the presence of OXA-48 in combination with other carbapenemases may often bias the interpretation of the DMDT. Third, the presence of OXA-48 cannot be detected by the DMDT even when no other carbapenemases are present and the use of the LFA rules out this limitation.

In practical terms, the superiority of the LFA is overwhelming. It is much easier to perform than the DMDT and gives results in 15 min for the five major carbapenemases. Of note, the DMDT provides results after 18–24 h of incubation.

Josa et al. showed that LFAs outweigh phenotypic boronic acid and EDTA synergy tests in carbapenemase detection and differentiation for Enterobacterales and *P. aeruginosa*. That is expected since the synergy tests can only detect MBLs, with no discrimination among them, and KPCs, but not OXA-48-like carbapenemases or any combination of them. Additionally, they may present false-positive results as EDTA may affect membrane permeability and boronic acid may increase the zone of inhibition of meropenem > 5 mm in case of AmpC hyper-production [27]. Sadek et al. found the K.N.I.V.O. Detection K-Set to have excellent performance, with 96.8% sensitivity and 100% specificity against a collection of 252 well-characterized Gram-negative strains. In this study, it succeeded in identifying KPC, NDM, IMP, VIM, and OXA-48-like carbapenemases with the exception of IMP-2, -8, -13, -19, which are mostly reported in Asian countries and only sporadically in Europe [28].

Carbapenem resistance is considered a public health issue of utmost importance as it is implicated in prolonged hospital stay and increased morbidity and mortality in hospitalized patients. The changing epidemiology and wide spread of different carbapenemases impedes their detection through culture-based methods, which are considered inadequate nowadays. Precision medicine practices, through the accurate identification of carbapenemases, are essential in order to promptly and efficiently apply infection control measures and therapeutics.

Carbapenemase-producing Gram-negative bacilli may occur by selective suppression on patient's flora, patient-to-patient transmission, or both. This, alongside plasmid transmission between species, makes them rapidly disseminate in the hospital environment and persist there as they are difficult to treat and eradicate. Considering the divergence of carbapenemases, speed and accuracy in their tracking is crucial in order to rapidly identify potential outbreaks, apply infection control measures to withhold their spread, and avoid unnecessary isolation.

Furthermore, in the past few years, new inhibitor/b-lactam combinations have been developed and are included in the current guidelines for the treatment of MDR Gram-negative bacteria [29], whereas their activity is dependent on their mechanisms of resistance. Therefore, knowing the exact type of the carbapenemase present is a prerequisite for the proper use of these molecules. For instance, ceftazidime–avibactam is active against extended spectrum β-lactamase producers, non-MBL carbapenem-resistant *P. aeruginosa*, KPC-producing carbapenem-resistant Enterobacterales, and OXA-48-producing carbapenem-resistant Enterobacterales, but not against MBL-producing Enterobacterales and MBL-producing *P. aeruginosa*. Furthermore, infections by carbapenem-resistant Gram-negative bacteria are associated with high mortality rates and thus the prompt administration of the proper antimicrobial regiment is crucial [30].

In conclusion, the characterization of specific carbapenemases is crucial and, therefore, the double synergy test, which is widely used in Greece, does not seem appropriate in an endemic and highly diverse environment such as ours. Thus, we also suggest that the local epidemiology should be taken into account when selecting the most suitable test for carbapenemase detection.

Knowledge of the local epidemiology plays an important role in the practical implementation of tests. For example, apart from carbapenemase-production, *P. aeruginosa* is known to show resistance to carbapenems due to porin defects and this can influence the interpretation of phenotypic tests. In our area, however, which is endemic for VIM-producing

P. aeruginosa, carbapenem resistance in this species is common due to carbapenemases; thus, carbapenem-resistant isolates resulting from porin defects alone are rare.

Even though we included only single patient isolates, no sequencing-based or other molecular epidemiology methods were employed to better characterize the molecular epidemiology of the isolates, since this was beyond the scope of this work. This is a limitation of our work because the possible presence of a multi-drug-resistant clone in our collection (especially regarding VIM-producing *P. aeruginosa*) cannot be definitely excluded. Another limitation is that we only employed a molecular "gold-standard" method for the isolates that presented discrepancies between the results of the phenotypic methods and the LFA. Indeed, in some Enterobacterales in our collection (4/14) that were tested with the molecular technique, the Antimicrobial Resistance Direct Flow Chip detected the presence of bla_{NDM}, whereas the respective LFA result was negative for the NDM carbapenemase, indicating that the LFA lacks sensitivity as compared with the molecular gold standard. Our results are indicative of the performance of a single LFA kit and should not be generalized for all other available kits. Therefore, we would like to recommend the evaluation of LFAs for carbapenemase detection before their implementation in clinical practice.

4. Materials and Methods

4.1. Study Design

A total of 210 carbapenem-resistant Gram-negative bacteria (Enterobacterales and *P. aeruginosa*) were tested in parallel using the double meropenem disc-test [31] and the Carbapenem-Resistant K.N.I.V.O. Detection K-Set (Goldstream, Beijing Gold Mountain river Tech Development Co., Ltd., Beijing, China) immunochromatographic lateral flow assay. The isolates were recovered from patients hospitalized in AHEPA University Hospital between September 2021 and September 2022. Bacterial identification and antimicrobial susceptibility testing were performed using the automated system VITEK2 (bioMérieux, Marcy l'Etoile, France). Susceptibility testing results were interpreted according to the EUCAST breakpoints v 12.0 (2022). All isolates were tested phenotypically for the detection of MBL, KPC, or both carbapenemase categories using the meropenem disc test. Based on our hospital's epidemiology, MBL-positive *K. pneumoniae* were considered as probable VIM or NDM producers [32]. Therefore, MBL-positive *K. pneumoniae* isolates were further tested with the modified Hodge test [33]. In case of a negative Hodge test result, the isolate was considered as a probable NDM producer and was further tested using PCR for the detection of the bla_{NDM} gene. In cases of DMDT double positivity (positive for both MBL and KPC), the Hodge test was not performed for distinguishing VIM and NDM because it would be influenced by the presence of KPC. According to the local epidemiology, MBL-positive *P. mirabilis* and *P. aeruginosa* were deemed to be probable VIM producers [34,35] and were not tested further using the Hodge test or PCR. The discrepancies between the phenotypic tests and the LFA were resolved using the Antimicrobial Resistance Direct Flow Chip (AMR): a microarray-based molecular diagnostic assay (Master Diagnóstica Granada, Spain). This molecular assay is able to detect KPC, NDM, IMP, various OXA-type carbapenemases, GES, GIM, NMC/IMI, SME, SIM, CMY, DHA, CTX, SHV, and SIM β-lactamases.

4.2. Double Meropenem Disc Test

The double meropenem disc test is a disc test where four meropenem discs are used with and without carbapenemase inhibitors (EDTA and phenylboronic acid) [31]. First, a 0.5 McFarland bacterial suspension was prepared and bacteria were inoculated onto a Mueller Hinton agar plate. The meropenem discs were placed on the surface of the agar preferably in a cross-like formation. The first disc was left without inhibitors. In total, 10 μL of EDTA 0.1 M were added on the second and 20 μL (20 g/L) of phenylboronic acid were added on the third disc. On the fourth disc, both inhibitors were applied. The evaluation of the results was performed after 18–24 h of incubation as follows: No inhibition zone around the first disc or an inhibition zone with a diameter of <22 mm for Enterobacterales or <14 mm for *P. aeruginosa* is indicative of carbapenem resistance. An inhibition zone around the second and the fourth disc with a diameter ≥ 5 mm that of the first disc indicates MBL production. An inhibition zone around the third and the fourth disc with a diameter ≥ 5 mm that of the first disc indicates KPC production. An inhibition halo around the second and third disc with a diameter ≥ 5 mm that of the first disc and an even larger halo around the fourth disc indicates simultaneous MBL and KPC production.

In our area, where many carbapenemase-encoding genes are endemic and carbapenem resistance is common due to the presence of carbapenemases, we usually consider a test negative when no carbapenemase is present. In such cases, the inhibition zone around the discs is larger than the breakpoint used and no further testing is needed. In the present work, the term "indeterminate" was used for tests where, despite the presence of carbapenem resistance, no information about the type of carbapenemase(s) present could be obtained. This commonly happens in the presence of OXA-type carbapenemases and further testing is needed.

Of note, EDTA can have intrinsic activity against bacteria by disrupting their cell wall and this can sometimes result in inhibition diameters larger than 5 mm for the EDTA-containing discs. To detect this, a negative control can be used by placing a blank disc with EDTA only. In this work, blank discs were not applied because the test has been used for many years in our lab and we have noticed that this property of EDTA does not influence the interpretation of results among our isolates that may carry specific carbapenemase-encoding genes, especially when these are not OXA-type carbapenemase determinants.

4.3. Modified Hodge Test

The modified Hodge test [36] was performed by inoculating the study isolate together with a carbapenem-susceptible indicator strain (*E. coli* ATCC 25922). Briefly, a 0.5 McFarland suspension of the indicator strain was inoculated onto a Mueller Hinton agar plate with a sterile cotton swab. Thereafter, a carbapenem disc was placed at the center of the plate. In total, 3–5 colonies of the test isolate were streaked from the center to the periphery of the plate. After incubation for 18–24 h, the presence of a distorted inhibition zone due to growth of the indicator strain toward the carbapenem disc because of carbapenemase production of the study isolate was interpreted as a positive result.

4.4. Detection of bla_{NDM} by PCR

The bla_{NDM} gene was detected by PCR as previously reported [37]. This method was applied for MBL-positive and Hodge-test-negative *K. pneumoniae* isolates, as identified via phenotypic methods. The primers used were NDM-Fm (5′-GGTTTGGCGATCTGGTTTTC-3′) and NDM-Rm (5′-CGGAATGGCTCATCACGATC-3′). The thermal cycling conditions used were 10 min at 94 °C; 36 cycles for 30 s at 94 °C, 40 s at 52 °C, and 50 s at 72 °C; concluding with 5 min at 72 °C for the final extension.

4.5. Carbapenem-Resistant K.N.I.V.O. Detection K-Set

The Carbapenem-Resistant K.N.I.V.O. Detection K-Set (Goldstream, Beijing Gold Mountain river Tech Development Co., Ltd.) is a multiplex lateral immunochromatographic flow assay that directly identifies carbapenemases from a bacterial colony. The assay consists of two cassettes: A and B. Cassette A includes specific areas for the detection of VIM and OXA-48, whereas cassette B includes areas for IMP, KPC, and NDM detection. Both cassettes include a specific control (C) area. In case the control line does not appear, the test result should be considered invalid. If only one line appears in the control region, the sample is considered negative since it does not contain any carbapenemase or may contain carbapenemase(s) at a non-detectable level. The result is interpreted as positive if the red line appears in the control region and one or several lines appear in the VIM, O48 (OXA-48), IMP, KPC, and NDM test regions. The intensity of the red test lines may vary; thus, a weak line still indicates a positive result since it may represent cases of lower enzyme expression. The assay was performed according to the manufacturer's instructions. In total, 2–3 single isolated colonies of the isolate to be tested were collected from the plate with an inoculation loop and were resuspended in an Eppendorf tube containing the five drops of sample treatment solution included in the kit. Subsequently, 50 μL of the mixture were added horizontally into the sample well of each cassette. The results were interpreted visually after 10–15 min of incubation at room temperature.

4.6. Statistical Analysis

The Kappa coefficient of agreement was applied to assess the level of agreement between the DMDT and the LFA results in Enterobacterales and in *P. aeruginosa* isolates using SPSS 28.0.

5. Conclusions

The Carbapenem-Resistant K.N.I.V.O. Detection K-Set was equivalent to the standard procedures used in our lab for the detection of carbapenamases; however, it was much faster since it provided results in 15 min compared to a minimum of 24 h the aforementioned methods. Therefore, it is a valuable tool in the early implementation of appropriate antimicrobial therapy and infection control measures.

Supplementary Materials: The following supporting information can be downloaded at: https://www.mdpi.com/article/10.3390/antibiotics12040771/s1, Table S1: Carbapenem-resistant Enterobacterales tested for carbapenemase production using the double meropenem disc test (DMDT), the Hodge test, the PCR for NDM, and the lateral flow assay (LFA); Table S2: Carbapenem-resistant *P. aeruginosa* isolates tested for carbapenemase production using the double meropenem disc test (DMDT) and the lateral flow assay (LFA).

Author Contributions: A.T. contributed to data acquisition and interpretation, and drafted the manuscript. G.M. contributed to design, data acquisition and interpretation, drafted the manuscript and critically revised the manuscript. P.M. contributed to data acquisition and interpretation. A.K. contributed to data acquisition and data curation. C.K. contributed to data acquisition. A.D. contributed to data acquisition. L.K. contributed to data acquisition. L.S. contributed to supervision, interpretation and critically revised the manuscript. E.P. contributed to conception, supervision, drafted the manuscript and critically revised the manuscript. All authors have read and agreed to the published version of the manuscript.

Funding: This research received no external funding.

Institutional Review Board Statement: The publication of the results was approved by the AHEPA University Hospital bioethics committee (protocol number: 36129/05.07.2022).

Informed Consent Statement: Not applicable.

Data Availability Statement: The data presented in this study are available in the article and the supplementary material.

Acknowledgments: Not applicable.

Conflicts of Interest: The authors declare no conflict of interest.

References

1. Alfei, S.; Schito, A.M. β-lactam antibiotics and β-lactamase enzymes inhibitors, part 2: Our limited resources. *Pharmaceuticals* **2022**, *15*, 476. [CrossRef] [PubMed]
2. Meletis, G. Carbapenem resistance: Overview of the problem and future perspectives. *Ther. Adv. Infect. Dis.* **2016**, *3*, 15–21. [CrossRef]
3. Tzouvelekis, L.S.; Markogiannakis, A.; Psichogiou, M.; Tassios, P.T.; Daikos, G.L. Carbapenemases in Klebsiella pneumoniae and other Enterobacteriaceae: An evolving crisis of global dimensions. *Clin. Microbiol. Rev.* **2012**, *25*, 682–707. [CrossRef] [PubMed]
4. Meletis, G.; Exindari, M.; Vavatsi, N.; Sofianou, D.; Diza, E. Mechanisms responsible for the emergence of carbapenem resistance in Pseudomonas aeruginosa. *Hippokratia* **2012**, *16*, 303–307. [PubMed]
5. Partridge, S.R.; Kwong, S.M.; Firth, N.; Jensen, S.O. Mobile genetic elements associated with antimicrobial resistance. *Clin. Microbiol. Rev.* **2018**, *31*, e00088-17. [CrossRef] [PubMed]
6. Castanheira, M.; Simner, P.J.; Bradford, P.A. Extended-spectrum β-lactamases: An update on their characteristics, epidemiology and detection. *JAC Antimicrob. Resist.* **2021**, *3*, dlab092. [CrossRef] [PubMed]

7. Ambler, R.P. The structure of beta-lactamases. *Philos. Trans. R. Soc. Lond. B Biol. Sci.* **1980**, *289*, 321–331.
8. Queenan, A.M.; Bush, K. Carbapenemases: The versatile beta-lactamases. *Clin. Microbiol. Rev.* **2007**, *20*, 440–458. [CrossRef]
9. Poirel, L.; Pitout, J.D.; Nordmann, P. Carbapenemases: Molecular diversity and clinical consequences. *Future Microbiol.* **2007**, *2*, 501–512. [CrossRef]
10. Nordmann, P.; Cuzon, G.; Naas, T. The real threat of Klebsiella pneumoniae carbapenemase-producing bacteria. *Lancet Infect. Dis.* **2009**, *9*, 228–236. [CrossRef]
11. Rapp, R.P.; Urban, C. Klebsiella pneumoniae carbapenemases in Enterobacteriaceae: History, evolution, and microbiology concerns. *Pharmacotherapy* **2012**, *32*, 399–407. [CrossRef] [PubMed]
12. Walther-Rasmussen, J.; Høiby, N. OXA-type carbapenemases. *J. Antimicrob. Chemother.* **2006**, *57*, 373–383. [CrossRef] [PubMed]
13. Walsh, T.R.; Toleman, M.A.; Poirel, L.; Nordmann, P. Metallo-beta-lactamases: The quiet before the storm? *Clin. Microbiol. Rev.* **2005**, *18*, 306–325. [CrossRef] [PubMed]
14. Zhao, W.H.; Hu, Z.Q. IMP-type metallo-β-lactamases in Gram-negative bacilli: Distribution, phylogeny, and association with integrons. *Crit. Rev. Microbiol.* **2011**, *37*, 214–226. [CrossRef] [PubMed]
15. Zhao, W.H.; Hu, Z.Q. Epidemiology and genetics of VIM-type metallo-β-lactamases in Gram-negative bacilli. *Future Microbiol.* **2011**, *6*, 317–333. [CrossRef] [PubMed]
16. Nordmann, P.; Poirel, L.; Walsh, T.R.; Livermore, D.M. The emerging NDM carbapenemases. *Trends Microbiol.* **2011**, *19*, 588–595. [CrossRef] [PubMed]
17. Quale, J.; Bratu, S.; Gupta, J.; Landman, D. Interplay of efflux system, ampC, and oprD expression in carbapenem resistance of Pseudomonas aeruginosa clinical isolates. *Antimicrob. Agents Chemother.* **2006**, *50*, 1633–1641. [CrossRef] [PubMed]
18. Poirel, L.; Potron, A.; Nordmann, P. OXA-48-like carbapenemases: The phantom menace. *J. Antimicrob. Chemother.* **2012**, *67*, 1597–1606. [CrossRef] [PubMed]
19. Girlich, D.; Poirel, L.; Nordmann, P. Value of the modified Hodge test for detection of emerging carbapenemases in Enterobacteriaceae. *J. Clin. Microbiol.* **2012**, *50*, 477–479. [CrossRef] [PubMed]
20. Tamma, P.D.; Simner, P.J. Phenotypic detection of carbapenemase-producing organisms from clinical isolates. *J. Clin. Microbiol.* **2018**, *56*, e01140-18. [CrossRef]
21. Boutal, H.; Moguet, C.; Pommiès, L.; Simon, S.; Naas, T.; Volland, H. The revolution of lateral flow assay in the field of AMR detection. *Diagnostics* **2022**, *12*, 1744. [CrossRef] [PubMed]
22. Bernabeu, S.; Bonnin, R.A.; Dortet, L. Comment on: Comparison of three lateral flow immunochromatographic assays for the rapid detection of KPC, NDM, IMP, VIM and OXA-48 carbapenemases in Enterobacterales. *J. Antimicrob. Chemother.* **2023**, *78*, 314–317. [CrossRef] [PubMed]
23. Hemwaranon, P.; Srisrattakarn, A.; Lulitanond, A.; Tippayawat, P.; Tavichakorntrakool, R.; Wonglakorn, L.; Daduang, J.; Chanawong, A. Recombinase Polymerase Amplification Combined with Lateral Flow Strip for Rapid Detection of OXA-48-like Carbapenemase Genes in Enterobacterales. *Antibiotics* **2022**, *11*, 1499. [CrossRef]
24. Vasilakopoulou, A.; Karakosta, P.; Vourli, S.; Kalogeropoulou, E.; Pournaras, S. Detection of KPC, NDM and VIM-Producing Organisms Directly from Rectal Swabs by a Multiplex Lateral Flow Immunoassay. *Microorganisms* **2021**, *9*, 942. [CrossRef]
25. Mendez-Sotelo, B.J.; López-Jácome, L.E.; Colín-Castro, C.A.; Hernández-Durán, M.; Martínez-Zavaleta, M.G.; RiveraBuendía, F.; Velázquez-Acosta, C.; Rodríguez-Zulueta, A.P.; MorfínOtero, M.d.R.; Franco-Cendejas, R. Comparison of Lateral Flow Immunochromatography and Phenotypic Assays to PCR for the Detection of CarbapenemaseProducing Gram-Negative Bacteria, a Multicenter Experience in Mexico. *Antibiotics* **2023**, *12*, 96. [CrossRef]
26. Meletis, G.; Vavatsi, N.; Exindari, M.; Protonotariou, E.; Sianou, E.; Haitoglou, C.; Sofianou, D.; Pournaras, S.; Diza, E. Accumulation of carbapenem resistance mechanisms in VIM-2-producing Pseudomonas aeruginosa under selective pressure. *Eur. J. Clin. Microbiol. Infect. Dis.* **2014**, *33*, 253–258. [CrossRef]
27. Josa, M.D.; Leal, R.; Rojas, J.; Torres, M.I.; Cortés-Muñoz, F.; Esparza, G.; Reyes, L.F. Comparative evaluation of phenotypic synergy tests versus RESIST-4 O.K.N.V. and NG Test Carba 5 lateral flow immunoassays for the detection and differentiation of carbapenemases in Enterobacterales and Pseudomonas aeruginosa. *Microbiol. Spectr.* **2022**, *10*, e01080-21. [CrossRef]
28. Sadek, M.; Bouvier, M.; Kerbol, A.; Poirel, L.; Nordmann, P. Evaluation of novel immunological rapid test (K.N.I.V.O. Detection K-Set) for rapid detection of carbapenemase producers in multidrug-resistant gram negatives. *Diagn. Microbiol. Infect. Dis.* **2022**, *104*, 115761. [CrossRef] [PubMed]
29. Lawandi, A.; Yek, C.; Kadri, S.S. IDSA guidance and ESCMID guidelines: Complementary approaches toward a care standard for MDR Gram-negative infections. *Clin. Microbiol. Infect.* **2022**, *28*, 465–469. [CrossRef]
30. Tamma, P.D.; Goodman, K.E.; Harris, A.D.; Tekle, T.; Roberts, A.; Taiwo, A.; Simner, P.J. Comparing the outcomes of patients with carbapenemase-producing and non-carbapenemase-producing carbapenem-resistant Enterobacteriaceae bacteremia. *Clin. Infect. Dis.* **2017**, *64*, 257–264. [CrossRef] [PubMed]
31. Tsakris, A.; Poulou, A.; Pournaras, S.; Voulgari, E.; Vrioni, G.; Themeli-Digalaki, K.; Petropoulou, D.; Sofianou, D. A simple phenotypic method for the differentiation of metallo-b-lactamases and class A KPC carbapenemases in Enterobacteriaceae clinical isolates. *J. Antibicrob. Chemother.* **2010**, *65*, 1664–1671. [CrossRef] [PubMed]
32. Protonotariou, E.; Meletis, G.; Pilalas, D.; Mantzana, P.; Tychala, A.; Kotzamanidis, C.; Papadopoulou, D.; Papadopoulos, T.; Polemis, M.; Metallidis, S.; et al. Polyclonal endemicity of carbapenemase-producing Klebsiella pneumoniae in ICUs of a Greek tertiary care hospital. *Antibiotics* **2022**, *11*, 149. [CrossRef] [PubMed]

33. Pasteran, F.; Veliz, O.; Rapoport, M.; Guerriero, L.; Corso, A. Sensitive and specific modified Hodge test for KPC and metallo-beta-lactamase detection in Pseudomonas aeruginosa by use of a novel indicator strain, Klebsiella pneumoniae ATCC 700603. *J. Clin. Microbiol.* **2011**, *49*, 4301–4303. [CrossRef]
34. Karampatakis, T.; Antachopoulos, C.; Tsakris, A.; Roilides, E. Molecular epidemiology of carbapenem-resistant Pseudomonas aeruginosa in an endemic area: Comparison with global data. *Eur. J. Clin. Microbiol. Infect. Dis.* **2018**, *37*, 1211–1220. [CrossRef]
35. Protonotariou, E.; Poulou, A.; Politi, L.; Meletis, G.; Chatzopoulou, F.; Malousi, A.; Metallidis, S.; Tsakris, A.; Skoura, L. Clonal outbreak caused by VIM-4-producing Proteus mirabilis in a Greek tertiary-care hospital. *Int. J. Antimicrob. Agents* **2020**, *56*, 106060. [CrossRef] [PubMed]
36. Clinical and Laboratory Standards Institute. *Performance Standards for Antimicrobial Susceptibility Testing: 19th Informational Supplement*; CLSI document M100–SClinical and Laboratory Standards Institute: Wayne, PA, USA, 2011.
37. Nordmann, P.; Poirel, L.; Carrër, A.; Toleman, M.A.; Walsh, T.R. How to detect NDM-1 producers. *J. Clin. Microbiol.* **2011**, *49*, 718–721. [CrossRef]

antibiotics

MDPI

Article

Identification of Efflux Pump Mutations in *Pseudomonas aeruginosa* from Clinical Samples

Sonia Quddus [1], Zainab Liaqat [1], Sadiq Azam [1], Mahboob Ul Haq [2], Sajjad Ahmad [3,4,*], Metab Alharbi [5] and Ibrar Khan [1,*]

1 Centre of Biotechnology and Microbiology, University of Peshawar, Peshawar 25120, Pakistan
2 Department of Pharmacy, Abasyn University, Peshawar 25000, Pakistan
3 Department of Computer Science and Physics, Center for Soft Matter and Biological Physics, Virginia Tech, Blacksburg, VA 24060, USA
4 Department of Health and Biological Sciences, Abasyn University, Peshawar 25000, Pakistan
5 Department of Pharmacology and Toxicology, College of Pharmacy, King Saud University, P.O. Box 2455, Riyadh 11451, Saudi Arabia
* Correspondence: sajjademaan8@gmail.com (S.A.); ibrarkhan1984@uop.edu.pk (I.K.)

Abstract: Efflux pumps are a specialized tool of antibiotic resistance used by *Pseudomonas aeruginosa* to expel antibiotics. The current study was therefore conducted to examine the expression of MexAB-OprM and MexCD-OprJ efflux pump genes. In this study, 200 samples were collected from Khyber Teaching Hospital (KTH) and Hayatabad Medical Complex (HMC) in Peshawar, Pakistan. All the isolates were biochemically identified by an Analytical Profile Index kit and at the molecular level by Polymerase Chain Reaction (PCR) utilizing specific primers for the OprL gene. A total of 26 antibiotics were tested in the current study using the guidelines of the Clinical and Laboratory Standard Institute (CLSI) and high-level resistance was shown to amoxicillin-clavulanic acid (89%) and low-level to chloramphenicol (1%) by the isolates. The antibiotic-resistant efflux pump genes MexA, MexB, OprM, MexR, MexC, MexD, OprJ, and NfxB were detected in 178 amoxicillin-clavulanic acid-resistant isolates. Mutations were detected in MexA, MexB, and OprM genes but no mutation was found in the MexR gene as analyzed by I-Mutant software. Statistical analysis determined the association of antibiotics susceptibility patterns by ANOVA: Single Factor $p = 0.05$. The in silico mutation impact on the protein structure stability was determined via the Dynamut server, which revealed the mutations might increase the structural stability of the mutants. The docking analysis reported that MexA wild protein showed a binding energy value of −6.1 kcal/mol with meropenem and the mexA mutant (E178K) value is −6.5 kcal/mol. The mexB wild and mutant binding energy value was −5.7 kcal/mol and −8.0 kcal/mol, respectively. Efflux pumps provide resistance against a wide range of antibiotics. Determining the molecular mechanisms of resistance in *P. aeruginosa* regularly will contribute to the efforts against the spread of antibiotic resistance globally.

Keywords: *Pseudomonas aeruginosa*; antibiotic-resistant efflux pump genes; nosocomial pathogen; antibiotics susceptibility pattern

1. Introduction

Pseudomonas aeruginosa is a predominant Gram-negative, aerobic, motile rod belonging to the family Pseudomonadaceae [1]. *P. aeruginosa* is present in soil and water and is a well-known pathogen causing diseases in humans, animals, and plants. Due to pigment production, pyoverdine, pyocyanin, and pyorubin by *P. aeruginosa* are easily detected on agar plates [2]. In comparison to other bacteria, the genome size of *P. aeruginosa* is very large (5.5–7 Mbp) and encodes many regulatory proteins/enzymes important for metabolism, development, and efflux system (hence for antibiotic resistance). Due to this huge encoding ability, *P. aeruginosa* becomes more stable and adapts to a variety of harsh environments [3]. *P. aeruginosa* is ubiquitous and causes severe infections in immunocompromised individuals. It causes healthcare-associated infections including sepsis, respiratory tract infections, hospital-acquired pneumonia, urinary tract infections, skin infections, bacterial keratitis, bacterial colitis, and otitis externa [4]. The treatment for the infections caused by *P. aeruginosa* includes mono and combination therapy [5]. The combination therapy may reduce the mortality rate in patients infected with *P. aeruginosa*. However, the well-documented antibiotic-resistant mechanisms of *P. aeruginosa* to a wide range of antibiotics are the main hurdle in treatment. Moreover, the over and misuse of antibiotics are responsible for antibiotic resistance in *P. aeruginosa* which is often multidrug resistant. *P. aeruginosa* has developed resistance against major antibiotic families including β-lactams, aminoglycosides, quinolones, and carbapenem [6]. The resistance mechanisms include adaptive resistance, acquired resistance, and intrinsic resistance [7]. The formation of biofilm protects against many antibiotics and contributes to the adaptive resistance of *P. aeruginosa* [8]. The antibiotic resistance genes can be acquired from the environment by *P. aeruginosa* via horizontal gene transfer and mutations are further adding to the phenomenon of acquired resistance [9]. The overexpression of efflux pumps diminished outer membrane permeability, and the production of enzymes for inactivating antibiotics are the main contributors to the intrinsic resistance of *P. aeruginosa* [10]. The efflux pumps of the Resistant Nodulation Division (RND) family are among the main efflux pumps of *P. aeruginosa* which contribute to resistance to many antibiotics. The MexAB-OprM is the first efflux pump detected in *P. aeruginosa*, regulated by the *mexR* gene, and is able to expel a wide range of antibiotics such as β-lactams, fluoroquinolones, tetracycline, macrolides, β-lactamase inhibitors, chloramphenicol, and sulfonamides. The efflux pump MexCD-OprJ, regulated by the nfxB gene is similar to the MexAB-OprM efflux pump [11]. Other efflux pumps such as MexEF-OprN and MexXY-OprM show resistance to a narrower spectrum of antibiotics [12]. There is a need to investigate the role of efflux pumps in clinical isolates of *P. aeruginosa* so that appropriate strategies and antibiotics can be used to manage the respective diseases. The current study focused on the expression and mutations of MexAB-OprM and MexCD-OprJ efflux pumps in clinical isolates of *P. aeruginosa* and correlated the expression of genes with antibiotic susceptibility profiles of *P. aeruginosa*.

2. Materials and Methods

2.1. Isolation and Identification of Bacterial Isolates

The current research was carried out at the Molecular Microbiology laboratory of the Centre of Biotechnology and Microbiology (COBAM), University of Peshawar.

A total of 200 clinical samples of *P. aeruginosa* were collected, of which 52 were from the Pathology and Microbiology laboratory of Khyber Teaching Hospital (KTH) Peshawar and 148 from the Hayatabad Medical Complex (HMC) Peshawar. All the samples were inoculated on nutrient agar and MacConkey agar plates and were incubated at 37 °C for 24 h for bacterial growth. After incubation, bacterial colonies were subjected to phenotypic and genotypic identification. The phenotypic identification was carried out by Gram staining to determine the Gram-negative status of the bacteria [13]. For biochemical identification, Analytical Profile Index (API 20E) strips were used [14].

2.2. Extraction of Genomic DNA

After the identification of isolates, 24 h old bacterial cultures were used for the extraction of bacterial DNA via a GJC®DNA purification kit. After DNA extraction, DNA samples were run on 1.5% agarose gel and visualized under Bio-Rad Molecular Imager® Gel Doc™.

2.3. Molecular Identification of Bacterial Isolates

For confirmation of isolates, genotypic identification was performed via the *oprL* gene by using a specific primer under optimized PCR conditions (Table 1) After PCR, the PCR product was run on 1.5% agarose gel and visualized under Bio-Rad Molecular Imager® Gel Doc™.

Table 1. Primer sequences with optimized PCR conditions.

Gene	Primer	Product Size (bp)	Annealing Temperature (°C)
OprL	F ATGGAAATGCTGAAATTCGGC R CTTCTTCAGCTCGACGCGACG	504	55
MexA	F CTATGCAACGAACGCCAGC R AGCCCTTGCTGTCGGTTTTC	1152	56
MexB	F TAGGCCCATTTTCGCGTGG R CGGTACCCAGAAGATCGCC	3043	56
OprM	F CGGTCCTTCCTTTCCCTGG R CAAGCCTGGGGATCTTCCTT	1451	55
MexR	F CAAGCGGTTGCGCGG R CCCCGTGAATCCCGACCTG	425	56
MexC	F TTACTGTTGCGGCGCAGG R CGTGCAATAGGAAGGATCGG	1152	55
MexD	F CAGCAGCCAGACGAAACAGA R TTCTTCATCAAGCGGCCGAA	3066	56
OprJ	F CTGCCGCCTCGATGTACC R GTATCGGCGCTGCTGATCG	1412	55
NfxB	F GACCCTGATTTCCCATGACG R GGAACATCTGCTCCAGGGTAT	530	56

2.4. Antibiotic Susceptibility Testing

The antibiotic susceptibility pattern of the identified isolates was performed by the Kirby Bauer disc diffusion method against selected antibiotics (Table 2) as prescribed by the Clinical and Laboratory Standards Institute (CLSI) 2019. Sterile plates of Muller Hinton Agar (MHA) were prepared, and selected antibiotic discs were placed and incubated for 24 h at 37 °C. The zones of inhibition were measured and interpreted as susceptible, intermediate, and resistant according to the CLSI guidelines [15].

Table 2. List of antibiotics.

S. No	Antibiotics (μg)	Family (Symbol)
1	Amikacin (20)	Aminoglycoside (AK)
2	Gentamicin (10)	Aminoglycoside (CN)
3	Azithromycin (30)	Macrolide (AZM)
4	Tigecycline (15)	Tetracycline (TGC)
5	Chloramphenicol (30)	Chloramphenicol (C)
6	Ciprofloxacin (5)	Fluoroquinolone (CIP)
7	Levofloxacin (5)	Fluoroquinolone (LEV)
8	Moxifloxacin (5)	Fluoroquinolone (MXF)
9	Amoxicillin (25)	β-lactam (penicillin) (AML)
10	Amoxicillin-clavulanic acid (30)	β-lactam (penicillin) (AMC)
11	Piperacillin-tazobactam (110)	β-lactam (penicillin) (TZP)
12	Aztreonam (30)	β-lactam (monobactams) (ATM)
13	Cefotaxime (30)	β-lactam (cephalosporin) (CTX)
14	Cefepime (30)	β-lactam (cephalosporin) (FEP)
15	Ceftazidime (30)	β-lactam (cephalosporin) (CAZ)

Table 2. *Cont.*

S. No	Antibiotics (μg)	Family (Symbol)
16	Cefoperazone (75)	β-lactam (cephalosporin) (CFP)
17	Cefoperazone-sulbactam (105)	β-lactam (cephalosporin) (SCF)
18	Ceftriaxone (30)	β-lactam (cephalosporin) (CRO)
19	Cefixime (5)	β-lactam (cephalosporin) (CFM)
20	Meropenem (10)	β-lactam (carbapenem) (MEM)
21	Imipenem (10)	β-lactam (carbapenem) (IMP)
22	Fosfomycin (50)	Fosfomycin (FOS)
23	Colistin (10)	Polymyxin (CT)
24	Polymyxin B (300)	Polymyxin (PB)
25	Trimethoprim-sulfamethoxazole (25)	Sulfonamide (SXT)
26	Nitrofurantoin (300)	Nitrofurantoin (F)

2.5. Molecular Detection of Efflux Pump Resistance Genes

The efflux pump-resistant genes *MexA-MexB-OprM* and *MexC-MexD-OprJ*, with regulators *mexR* and *nfxB*, respectively, were investigated in all isolates by PCR. The PCR mixture was prepared by adding 12.5 μL GoTaq® Green Master Mix 2X, 1 μL upstream primer, 1 μL downstream primer, 25 μL PCR grade water, and 1 μL DNA template and run under optimized conditions (Table 1). After that, samples were run on 1.5% agarose gel and visualized under the gel documentation system.

2.6. Mutational Analysis of PCR Products

After the amplification of efflux pump-resistant genes, PCR products were sent to Macrogen for sequencing using the next-generation sequencing (NGS) method. The sequences of genes were analyzed through the BioEdit Sequence Alignment Editor Software (Borland, Vista, CA, USA). The consensus sequence of each gene was checked through the Basic Local Alignment Search Tool (BLAST) which checked the local similarity between the sequences. Interpretation of I-mutant results was used to predict either an increase or decrease in the function of the respective proteins.

2.7. Computational Studies

By using the Expasy translater tool (https://web.expasy.org/translate/ accessed on 8 September 2022), the nucleotide sequences of the genes were converted into amino acid sequences to be used for structure modeling and docking studies. The SWISS-MODEL server (https://swissmodel.expasy.org/) was used for the structural modeling of wild and mutant proteins. SWISS-MODEL accepts the protein sequence in FASTA format. The protein structure visualization was performed through UCSF Chimera v1.16 (http://www.cgl.ucsf.edu/chimera/ accessed on 15 September 2022). The mutation effect on the protein structure and overall conformational stability was determined by the Dynamut server available at https://biosig.lab.uq.edu.au/dynamut/prediction accessed on 20 September 2022. The PyRx 0.8 virtual screening software (https://pyrx.sourceforge.io/ accessed on 25 September 2022) was used for molecular docking studies to determine the intermolecular binding conformation of wild and mutant proteins with meropenem. The docking was performed on Intel® Core(TM) i5-3230M CPU @ 2.60 GHz with 64-bit Windows 8.1. The grid box dimensions were set manually to cover the whole protein. For mexA wild-type protein, the dimensions were x = 346.21 Å, y = 317.80 Å, and z = 333.04 Å. The docking dimensions for the mexA mutant were set to 74.19 Å on x = 342.03 Å, 282.35 Å on the *y*-axis, and 329.09 Å on the *z*-axis. The box dimensions for mexB wild were set to 79.64 Å on the *x*-axis, −45.72 Å on the *y*-axis, and −17.71 Å on the z-axis. For the mexB mutant, the dimensions used were x = −34.72 Å, *y*-axis = −22.56 Å, and *z*-axis = 20.64 Å. The docking complexes were analyzed by UCSF Chimera v1.16 and Discovery Studio (DS) Visualizer v2021.

2.8. Statistical Analysis

A chi-square analysis was conducted using SPSS version 20 to find the association between the expected value of *E. coli* with the observed $p \leq 0.05$. For that, the number of samples was (n) set at 150 and the degree of freedom was taken at n-1. For comparative analysis, one-way analysis of variance (ANOVA) among the continuous values of antibiotics with *P. aeruginosa* was performed and $p \leq 0.05$ values were considered statistically significant.

3. Results

The clinical isolates of *P. aeruginosa* were collected from the KTH and the HMC, Peshawar, from different sources: wound swab, urine, pus, blood, ear pus, and cerebrospinal fluid (Table 3). One hundred and eight patients (54%) were male and 92 (46%) were female and of different age groups. Among 200 isolates of *P. aeruginosa*, a high rate of prevalence was recorded in the age group of 21 to 30 (21.5%) followed by the age group of 31 to 40 (18.5%) (Table 4).

Table 3. Collection of clinical samples of *P. aeruginosa* from various sources.

Source	Number (Percentage)
Urine catheter	1 (0.5)
Stone analysis	1 (0.5)
Urine	28 (14)
Pus	57 (28.5)
Wound swab	94 (47)
Blood	7 (3.5)
Sputum	9 (4.5)
CSF	1 (0.5)
Ear swab	2 (1.0)
Total	200

Table 4. Frequency of patients' gender and age.

Parameter		Frequency	Percentage
Gender	Male	108	54.0
	Female	92	46.0
Age Group (Years)	1–10	12	6
	11–20	30	15
	21–30	43	21.5
	31–40	37	18.5
	41–50	23	11.5
	51–60	25	12.5
	61–70	21	10.5
	71–80	8	4
	81–90	1	0.5

3.1. Antibiotics Susceptibility Testing

The antibiotic sensitivity pattern of the isolates revealed sensitivity to AK, SCF, and TZP and high resistance to AMC, CTX, CFM, and SXT (Table 5)

Table 5. Antibiotic susceptibility pattern of *P. aeruginosa*.

Antibiotics	Resistant (*n*)	Percentage (%)	Intermediate (*n*)	Percentage (%)	Susceptible (*n*)	Percentage (%)
AK	40	20	4	2	156	78
CN	88	44	10	5	102	51
CIP	79	39.5	9	4.5	112	58
LEV	71	35.5	23	11.5	106	53
MXF	80	40	11	5.5	109	54.5
AML	6	3	-	-	1	0.5
AMC	178	89	1	0.5	21	10.5
TZP	49	24.5	5	2.5	146	73
ATM	71	35.5	16	8.0	113	56.5
CTX	128	64	5	2.5	67	33.5
FEP	72	36	7	3.5	121	60.5
CAZ	73	36.5	11	5.5	116	58
CEP	72	36	15	7.5	113	56.5
SCF	49	24.5	10	5.0	141	70.5
CRO	96	48	11	5.5	93	46.5
CFM	158	79	7	3.5	35	17.5
MEM	63	31.5	8	4.0	129	64.5
IMP	63	31.5	11	5.5	126	63
AZM	-	-	-	-	7	3.5
TGC	100	50	12	6	88	44
CT	62	31	17	8.5	121	60.5
PB	63	31.5	21	10.5	116	58
FOS	6	3	2	1	22	11
C	2	1	-	-	5	2.5
SXT	125	62.5	5	2.5	70	35
F	15	7.5	-	-	15	7.5

3.2. Molecular Detection of Efflux Pump Resistance Genes in Isolates of P. aeruginosa

The PCR results revealed the presence of efflux pump genes in *P. aeruginosa* isolates (Figures 1–8). By comparing the results of PCR with the antibiotic susceptibility pattern of isolates, it was concluded that efflux pump resistance genes were detected mostly among amoxicillin/clavulanic acid-resistant isolates (n = 178; 89%) (Table 6).

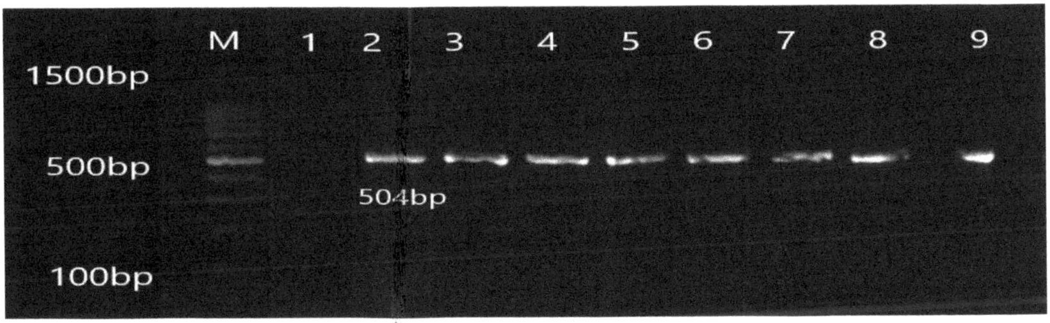

Figure 1. Electrophoresis showing amplicons of *P. aeruginosa mexB* gene. Lane M: 100 bp plus molecular marker, Lane 1: Negative control, Lane 2–9: Positive isolates of *mexB* gene.

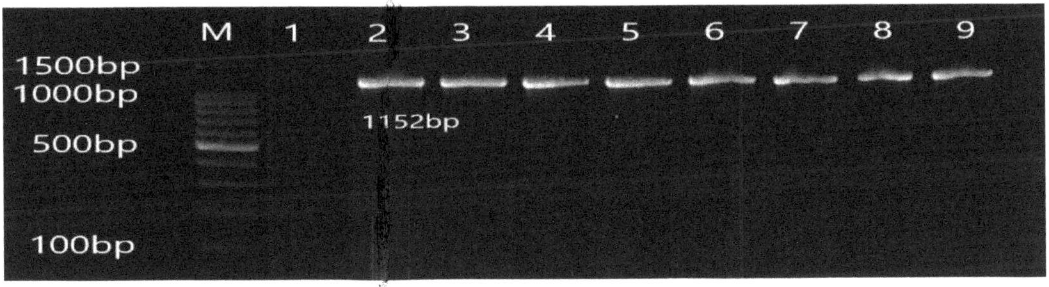

Figure 2. Electrophoresis showing amplicons of *P. aeruginosa mexA* gene. Lane M: 100 bp molecular marker, Lane 1: Negative control, Lane 2–9: Positive isolates of *mexA* gene.

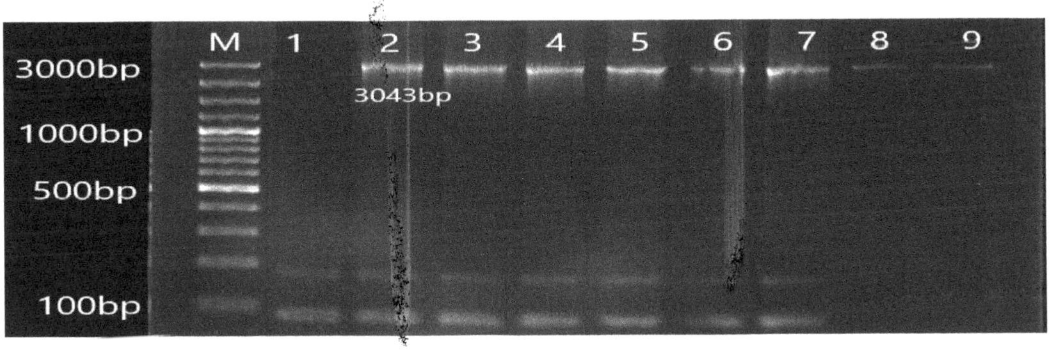

Figure 3. Electrophoresis showing amplicons of *P. aeruginosa oprL* gene. Lane M: 100 bp molecular marker, Lane 1: Negative control, Lane 2: Positive control, Lane 3–9: Positive isolates of *oprL*.

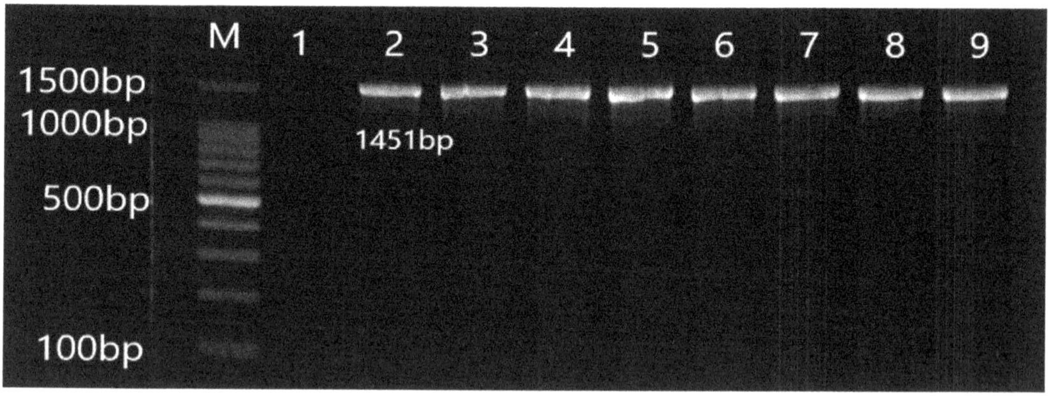

Figure 4. Electrophoresis showing amplicons of *P. aeruginosa mexC* gene. Lane M: 100 bp molecular marker, Lane 1: Negative control, Lane 2–9: Positive isolates of *mexC* gene.

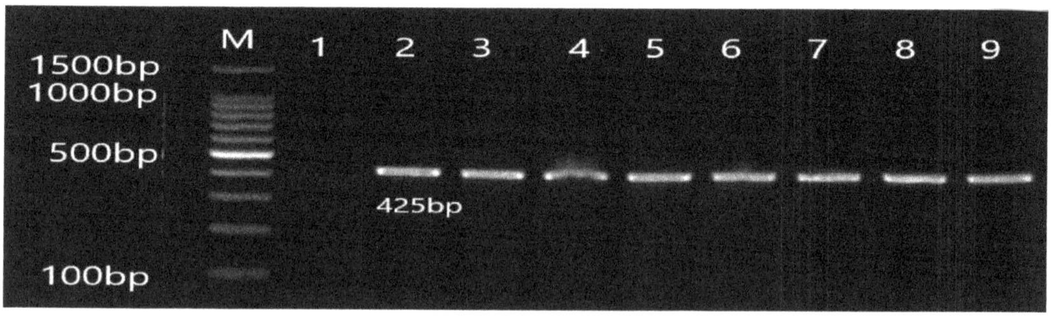

Figure 5. Electrophoresis showing amplicons of *P. aeruginosa mexR* gene. Lane M: 100 bp molecular marker, Lane 1: Negative control, Lane 2–9: Positive isolates of *mexR* gene.

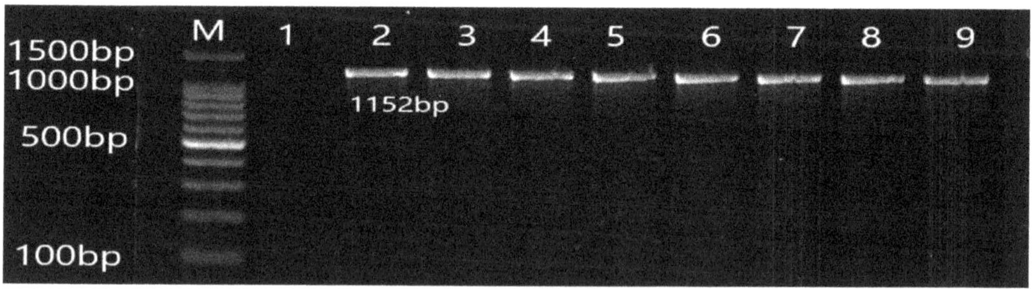

Figure 6. Electrophoresis showing amplicons of *P. aeruginosa oprM* gene. Lane M: 100 bp molecular marker, Lane 1: Negative control, Lane 2–9: Positive isolates of *oprM* gene.

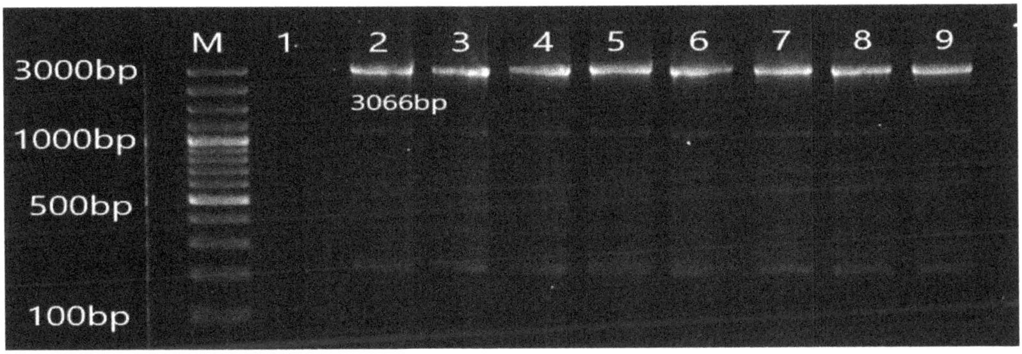

Figure 7. Electrophoresis showing amplicons of *P. aeruginosa mexD* gene. Lane M: 100 bp plus molecular marker, Lane 1: Negative control, Lane 2–9: Positive isolates of *mexD* gene.

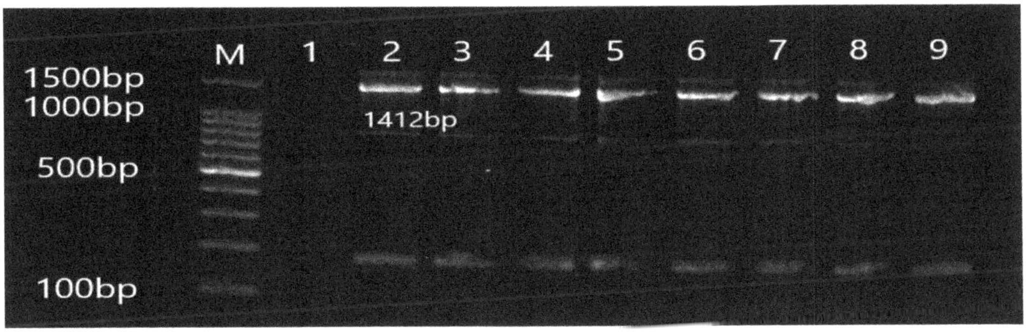

Figure 8. Electrophoresis showing amplicons of *P. aeruginosa oprJ* gene. Lane M: 100 bp molecular marker, Lane 1: Negative control, Lane 2–9: Positive isolates of *oprJ* gene.

Table 6. Polymerase chain reactions of Antibiotic resistance efflux pump genes.

Positive Isolates of Efflux Pump Genes	Genes	Positive Result
AMC-resistant isolates	*MexA*	178 (89%)
	MexB	178 (89%)
	OprM	178 (89%)
	MexR	178 (89%)
	MexC	178 (89%)
	MexD	178 (89%)
	OprJ	178 (89%)
	NfxB	178 (89%)

3.3. Mutational Analysis of Antibiotic-Resistant Efflux Pump Genes

The mutational analysis was performed for the *mexA*, *mexB*, *oprM*, and *mexR* genes. In the sequences of *mexA* (Tables 7 and 8), *mexB* (Tables 9 and 10), and *oprM* gene (Tables 11 and 12) mutations were detected while no mutation was detected in the *mexR* gene.

Table 7. Non-synonymous mutation of the *mexA* gene.

Codon Position	Reference Amino Acid	Altered Amino Acid	Amino Acid Position
389	GGT (Glycine)	AGT (Serine)	368

Table 8. *mexA* Prediction result of I-Mutant software.

Wild Type	New	I-Mutant Prediction Effect	DDG Value	Reliability Index (RI)	Temperature	pH
G (Glycine)	S (Serine)	Decrease	−1	8	25	7

Table 9. Synonymous and non-synonymous mutations of the mexB gene.

Codon Position	Reference Amino Acid Position	Altered Amino Acid Position	Amino Acid Position
	Synonymous mutation of *mexB* gene		
148	TCC-TCG	Serine	129
154	AGC-AGT	Serine	130
184	GTC-GTG	Valine	142
256	CCT-CCG	Proline	166
259	CTC-CTA	Leucine	167
302	AAA-AAG	Lysine	290
308	GTA-GTC	Valine	291
635	CAA-CAG	Glutamine	673
	Non-synonymous mutation of the *mexB* gene		
126	Asparagine (AAC)	Aspartate (GAC)	123
129	Tyrosine (TAT)	Asparagine (AAT)	124
136	Leucine (CTC)	Arginine (CGC)	126
138	Phenylalanine (TTC)	Tyrosine (TAC)	127
140	Phenylalanine (TTC)	Isoleucine (ATC)	128
151	Aspartate (GAC)	Glutamate (GAG)	131
165	Alanine (GCC)	Glycine (GGC)	136
167	Cysteine (TGC)	Serine (AGC)	137
170	Proline (CCG)	Methionine (ATG)	138
191	Glutamine (CAA)	Glutamate (GAA)	145
197	Leucine (CTC)	Glycine (GGC)	147
200	Proline (CCC)	Threonine (ACC)	148
203	Asparagine (AAC)	Aspartate (GAC)	149
215	Proline (CCC)	Alanine (GCC)	143
219	Leucine (CTG)	Glutamine (CAG)	154
228	Alanine (GCC)	Valine (GTG)	157
231	Leucine (CTC)	Glutamine (CAG)	158

Table 9. *Cont.*

Codon Position	Reference Amino Acid Position	Altered Amino Acid Position	Amino Acid Position
244	Histidine (CAC)	Glutamine (CAA)	162
269	Glutamine (CAA)	Glutamate (GAA)	171
283	Histidine (CAT)	Glutamine (CAG)	175
292	Histidine (CAC)	Arginine (CGG)	287
303	Serine (TCG)	Alanine (GCG)	291
321	Leucine (CTG)	Methionine (ATG)	296
324	Leucine (CTG)	Valine (GTG)	298
327	Leucine (CTG)	Valine (GTG)	299
330	Arginine (CGT)	Glycine (GGT)	300
340	Proline (CCT)	Valine (GTT)	302
365	Asparagine (AAC)	Lysine (AAG)	311
378	Histidine (CAC)	Asparagine (AAC)	316
388	Alanine (GCT)	Valine (GTT)	319
424	Alanine (GCC)	Glycine (GGC)	331
429	Cysteine (TGC)	Glycine (GGT)	333
439	Proline (CCG)	Glutamine (CAG)	336
441	Leucine (CTG)	Valine (GTG)	337
456	Histidine (CAC)	Tyrosine (TAC)	342
488	Asparagine (AAT)	Lysine (AAG)	472
536	Histidine (CAT)	Glutamine (CAG)	488
590	Asparagine (AAC)	Lysine (AAG)	506
599	Histidine (CAT)	Tyrosine (CAG)	509
732	Histidine (CAT)	Tyrosine (CAG)	673

Table 10. *MexB* gene Prediction results of I-Mutant software.

Wild Type	New Type	I-Mutant Prediction Effect	DDG Value	Reliability Index (RI)	Temperature	pH
N	D	Decrease	−0.95	7	25	7
Y	N	Increase	−0.24	0	25	7
L	R	Decrease	−0.95	7	25	7
F	Y	Decrease	−0.85	7	25	7
F	I	Decrease	−1.99	9	25	7
D	E	Decrease	−0.59	7	25	7
A	G	Decrease	−1.03	7	25	7
C	S	Decrease	−0.53	1	25	7
P	M	Decrease	−0.96	1	25	7
Q	E	Decrease	−0.29	4	25	7
L	G	Increase	0.22	2	25	7

Table 10. *Cont.*

Wild Type	New Type	I-Mutant Prediction Effect	DDG Value	Reliability Index (RI)	Temperature	pH
P	T	Decrease	−0.02	1	25	7
N	D	Increase	0.11	5	25	7
P	A	Decrease	−1.02	4	25	7
L	Q	Decrease	0.14	1	25	7
A	V	Decrease	−0.93	6	25	7
L	Q	Decrease	0.00	3	25	7
H	Q	Decrease	−0.61	7	25	7
Q	E	Decrease	−0.11	1	25	7
H	Q	Decrease	−0.61	7	25	7
H	R	Decrease	−1.37	9	25	7
S	A	Decrease	−0.90	8	25	7
L	M	Decrease	−0.80	5	25	7
L	V	Decrease	−1.30	6	25	7
L	V	Decrease	−1.32	6	25	7
R	G	Decrease	−0.48	1	25	7
P	V	Decrease	−1.57	4	25	7
N	K	Increase	−0.48	3	25	7
H	N	Decrease	−0.66	9	25	7
A	V	Decrease	−1.37	7	25	7
A	G	Increase	−0.51	1	25	7
C	G	Decrease	−0.76	0	25	7
P	Q	Decrease	−0.41	6	25	7
L	V	Decrease	−0.74	4	25	7
H	Y	Decrease	0.04	1	25	7
N	K	Increase	0.04	4	25	7
H	Q	Decrease	−0.53	6	25	7
N	K	Decrease	−0.55	2	25	7
H	Q	Decrease	−0.97	8	25	7
H	Q	Decrease	−0.91	6	25	7

Table 11. Synonymous and non-synonymous mutations of the *oprM* gene.

Codon Position	Reference Amino Acid Position	Altered Amino Acid Position	Amino Acid Position
	Non-synonymous mutation of the OprM gene		
11	Glutamine (CAA)	Arginine (CGC)	7
50	Valine (GTG)	Alanine (GCG)	20
	Synonymous mutation of the *OprM* gene		
43	ACT-ACC	T	17

Table 12. *OprM* gene Prediction results of I-Mutant software.

Wild Type	New Type	I-Mutant Prediction Effect	DDG Value	Reliability Index (RI)	Temperature	PH
Q (Glutamine)	R (Arginine)	Increase	−0.11	1	25	7
V (Valine)	A (Alanine)	Decrease	−1.66	8	25	7

3.4. Mutation Impact on Structure Stability

The impact of mutations on the thermodynamic characteristics of wild-type and mutant proteins was revealed through the Dynamut server. The Dynamut predicts each mutation's impact on protein conformational energy. As given in Table S1, the mutation effect determines the increased stability of mutant proteins compared to wild proteins. The E178K of mexA showed a destabilizing effect. In case of mexB, mutations such as R2T, W4T, L5V, D6T, P7F, A8E, N9Q, L10G, N11T, S12D, Y13P, Q14D, L15I, T16A, P17Q, G18V, D19Q, S21Q, S22N, A23K, I24L, H25Q, A26L, Q27A, N28T, V29P, Q30L, I31L, S32P, S33Q, G34E, Q35V, L36Q, G37R, G38Q, L39G, P40I, N43T, G44K, Q45A, H46V, L47K, A49F, T50L, I51M, I52V, G53V, K54G, T55V, R56V, L57S, Q58T, T59D, A60G, E61S, Q62M, F63T, E64K, N65E, I66D, L68S, K69N, V70Y, N71I, P72V, D73S, G74N, S75I, V77D, R78P, K80S, D81R, V82T, A83K, D84G, L87D, G88F, G89Q, H90V, D91F, Y92G, I94Q, N95Y, A96R, Q97S, F98M, N99R, G100I, S101W, P102L, G103D, V104P, R105A, Y106K, R107L, D108N, Q109S, and A110Y reported a destabilizing effect on the wild mexB protein. The vibrational entropy energy between the wild and mutant types was recorded in kcal/mol.

3.5. Docking Analysis

Molecular docking is a computational-based technique for intermolecular binding conformation. Here, the objective was to determine the mutation impact on meropenem drug binding with wild and mutant phenotypes of the genes. The docking results are provided in Table 13. The mexA wild protein complex binding energy value was −6.1 kcal/mol and the mexA mutant (E178K) value was −6.5 kcal/mol. The mexB wild protein complex binding energy value was −5.7 kcal/mol and the mexB mutant protein complex binding energy value was −8.0 kcal/mol. The binding conformation of meropenem with the mexA and mexB is shown in Figures 9 and 10.

Table 13. Docking energy score in kcal/mol.

Complex	Docking Score
max-A wild_meropenem	−6.1
max-A mutant (E178K) meropenem	−6.5
max-B wild_meropenem	−5.7
max-B mutant_meropenem	−8

Through discovery studio visualizer v2021 software, the binding interactions between protein and drug were determined. The wild-type MexA is involved in van der Waals and conventional hydrogen bonds with the drug, while the mutant formed van der Waals conventional hydrogen, and carbon-hydrogen bonds. The wild MexA active residue such as Arg35 is attached to the hydroxybutanal with the help of a conventional hydrogen bond while 1-azabicyclo[3.2.0]hept-2-ene of the drug produced chemical bonding with Ala40, Gly37, Ala 36, Gly99, Glu58, Lue96, Leu28, Leu24, Arg25, leu21, Phe61, Val64, and Ile75. In mutant MexA, Lys173 is attached to the 1-azabicyclo[3.2.0]hept-2-ene through a conventional hydrogen bond. The val175 is attached to the 1-azabicyclo[3.2.0]hept-2-ene with the help of a carbon-hydrogen bond. The active residues such as Pro176,Thr160, Ala177, Glu161, Phe165,Val 166,Ile158, Lys157, The174, Val125, Ile159, Val172, and Gly162 were engaged with 1-azabicyclo [3.2.0]hept-2-ene by Van der Waals bonding (Figure 11). In mexB wild, binding interactions involve Arg2 and Ile3 attached to the 1-azabicyclo[3.2.0]hept-

2-ene-2-carboxylic acid by a conventional hydrogen bond. The Asn28 is attached to the pyrrolidine-2-carboxamide chemical moiety via a conventional hydrogen bond. The active residues such as Pro17, Val20, Phe63, Ser21, Leu5, His25, Ile24, Arg56, Trp4, and Met1 interact with the drug by van der Waals interactions (Figure 12). The mexB mutant binding interactions involve Thr11, Gly10, and Phe7 with the pyrrolidine-2-carboxamide through conventional hydrogen bonding while Val5 is seen with 1-azabicyclo[3.2.0]hept-2-en-7-one. The active site residues Val42, Gln17, Ala16, Pro13, Glu8, Gln9, Thr208, Thr6, Ala45, Thr4, Lys44, Lys44, Thr43, and Val20 formed bonding to the protein via van der Waals interactions.

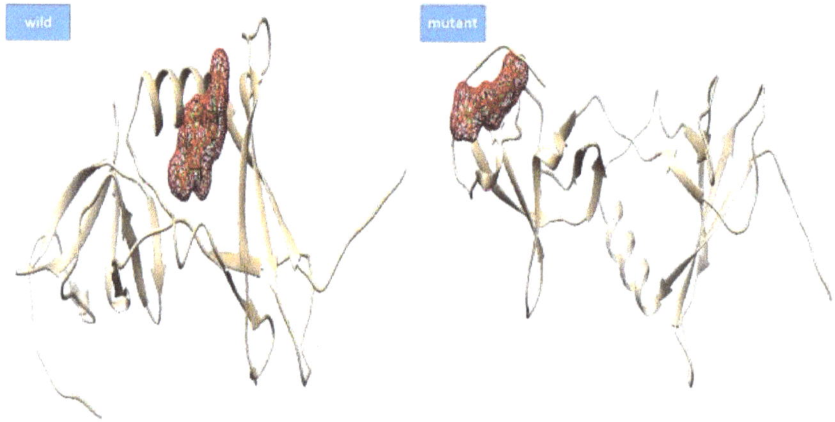

Figure 9. MexA wild and mutant intermolecular-docked complex with meropenem. The proteins are shown in tan cartoon style while the ligands are given in mesh.

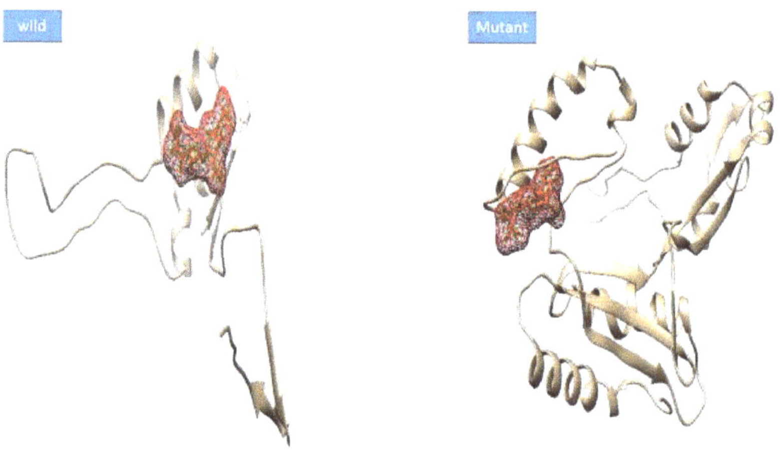

Figure 10. Binding conformation of meropenem with the mexB wild and mutant proteins. The proteins are shown in tan cartoon style while the ligands are given in mesh.

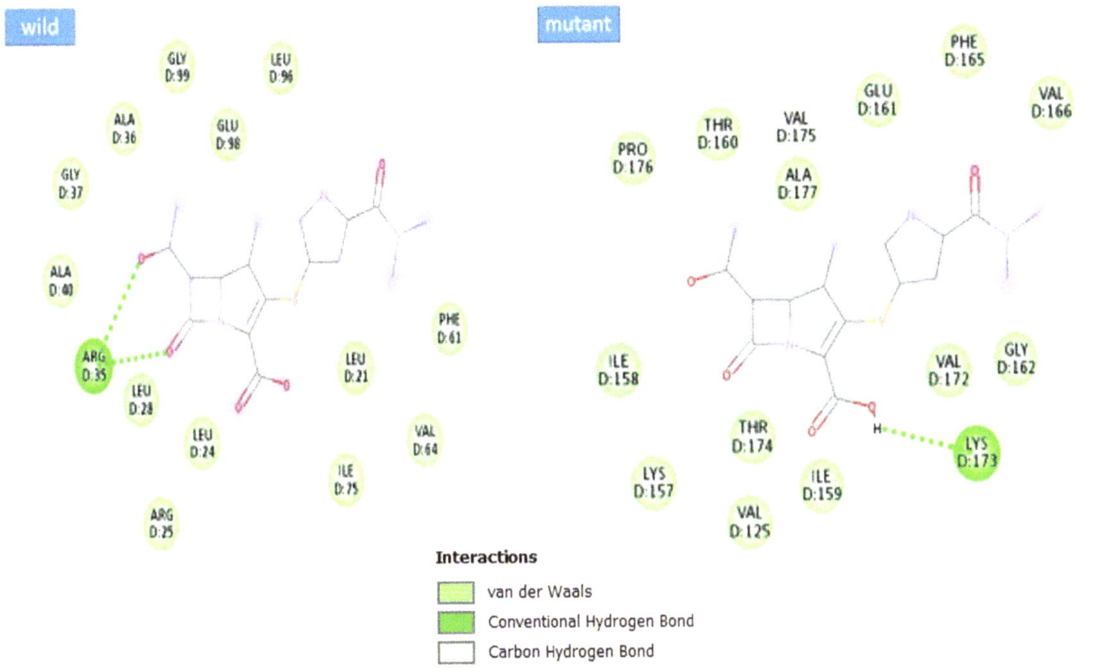

Figure 11. MexA wild and mutant binding interactions with meropenem. The compound is presented in a 2D line.

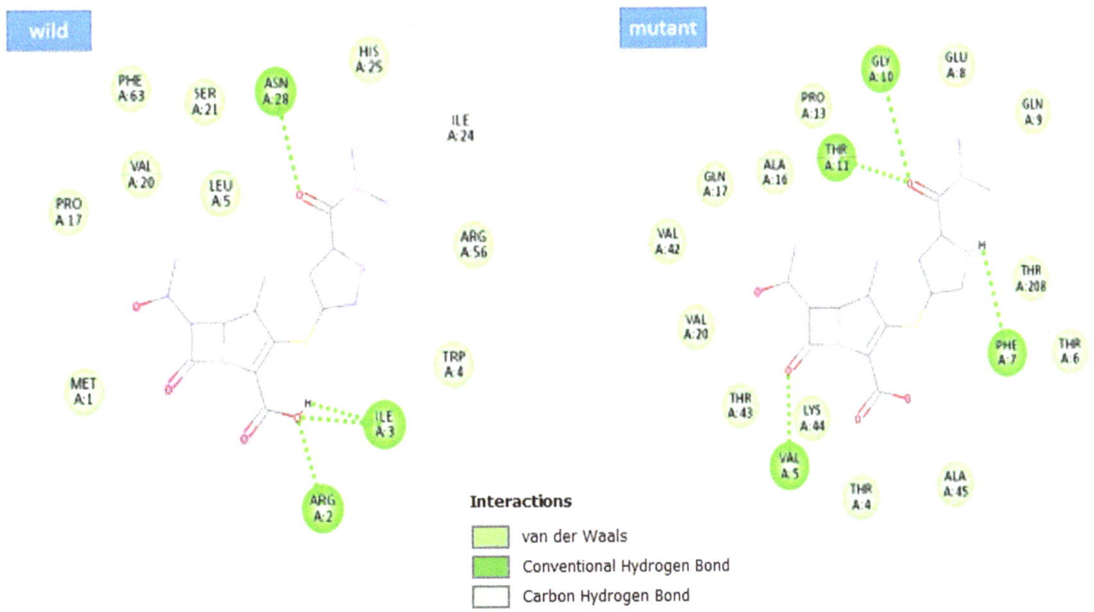

Figure 12. MexB wild and mutant binding interactions with meropenem. The compound is presented in a 2D line.

4. Discussion

A recent study investigated the expression of the *MexA* (88.2%) and *MexB* genes (70.5%) in 136 MDR and PDR isolates of *P. aeruginosa*. The study reported 69% *MexB* gene expression followed by 28.7% *MexC* expression, 43.4% *MexE* expression, and 74.6% *MexY* expression among isolates from the ICU. They were highly resistant to ticarcillin (80%), ciprofloxacin (74%), and meropenem (71%) [13].

In another study, antibiotic resistance-conferring efflux pumps were investigated in the isolates that were carbapenem-resistant (63.15%). The PCR results revealed overexpression in 19 (79.1%) isolates [14]. In the present study, MexAB-OprM and MexCD-OprJ efflux pumps were expressed in all the amoxicillin/clavulanic acid-resistant isolates. Mohseni et al., [15] investigated the efflux pumps conferring resistance among isolates collected from both human and animal sources. The PCR results showed an increased expression of the MexA gene as compared to the MexB gene. The isolates were 100% resistant to trimethoprim/sulfamethoxazole, cefazolin, ampicillin, kanamycin, and amoxicillin/clavulanic acid.

Efflux pump systems also mediate fluoroquinolone resistance in *P. aeruginosa*. In another study, out of 36 isolates, 88% were resistant to ofloxacin while 85% of them were resistant to sparfloxacin. Thus, the resistance mediated by efflux pump systems must be considered when introducing novel fluoroquinolones [16]. A study by Rudy et al. detected the expression of MexA-MexB-OprM efflux pump in 80% of isolates that were all ciprofloxacin resistant [17]. In the current study, 79 (39.5%) isolates were resistant to ciprofloxacin. The *MexA, MexB, OprM,* and *MexR* genes were detected in these ciprofloxacin-resistant isolates in accordance with the reported literature [18,19].

5. Conclusions

P. aeruginosa is known to adapt efficiently in harsh environments. All isolates in the present study were highly resistant to various families of antibiotics including beta-lactams, aminoglycosides, tetracycline, and carbapenems. Among 200 isolates, 178 were highly resistant and expressed all the selected efflux pump-resistant genes. For the better treatment of infections by *P. aeruginosa*, combination therapies may be a good choice to overcome the multidrug-resistant mechanisms of *P. aeruginosa*.

6. Future Recommendations

All isolates in the present study were highly resistant showing expression of efflux pumps. To overcome this hurdle, the implementation of efflux pump inhibitors with antibiotics would be helpful. Research for novel antibiotics and efflux pump inhibitors could be an interesting strategy for the better management of infections caused by *P. aeruginosa*.

Supplementary Materials: The following supporting information can be downloaded at: https://www.mdpi.com/article/10.3390/antibiotics12030486/s1, Table S1: Dynamut result of mexA and mexB.

Author Contributions: Conceptualization, I.K. and S.A. (Sajjad Ahmad); methodology, S.Q.; software, M.U.H., S.A. (Sadiq Azam); validation, I.K., S.A. (Sadiq Azam) and S.A. (Sajjad Ahmad); formal analysis, Z.L.; investigation, S.Q.; resources, M.A.; data curation, S.Q.; writing—original draft preparation, S.Q.; writing—review and editing, I.K., S.A. (Sadiq Azam), S.A. (Sajjad Ahmad); visualization, M.U.H.; supervision, I.K.; project administration, S.A. (Sajjad Ahmad); funding acquisition, M.A. All authors have read and agreed to the published version of the manuscript.

Funding: The authors express their gratitude to the Researchers Supporting Project number (RSP2023R462), King Saud University, Riyadh, Saudi Arabia.

Institutional Review Board Statement: Not required for our study.

Informed Consent Statement: Informed consent has been obtained from all the patients.

Data Availability Statement: The data generated in the research study is presented in the manuscript.

Conflicts of Interest: The authors declare no conflict of interest.

References

1. Peix, A.; Martha-Helena, B.; Encarna, V. Historical evolution and current status of the taxonomy of genus Pseudomonas. *Infect. Genet. Evol.* **2009**, *9*, 1132–1147. [CrossRef] [PubMed]
2. Meyer, J.M. Pyoverdines: Pigments, siderophores and potential taxonomic markers of fluorescent Pseudomonas species. *Arch. Microbiol.* **2000**, *174*, 135–142. [CrossRef] [PubMed]
3. Meliani, A. The multifactorial resistance of Pseudomonas aeruginosa. *EXCLI J.* **2020**, *19*, 813–816. [PubMed]
4. Streeter, K.; Katouli, M. Pseudomonas aeruginosa: A review of their Pathogenesis and Prevalence in Clinical Settings and the Environment. *Epidemiol. Infect.* **2016**, *2*, 25–32. [CrossRef]
5. El Solh, A.A.; Alhajhusain, A. Update on the treatment of Pseudomonas aeruginosa pneumonia. *J. Antimicrob. Chemother.* **2009**, *64*, 229–238. [CrossRef] [PubMed]
6. Hirsch, E.B.; Vincent, T.H. Impact of multidrug-resistant Pseudomonas aeruginosa infection on patient outcomes. *Expert Rev. Pharmacoecon. Outcomes Res.* **2010**, *10*, 441–451. [CrossRef] [PubMed]
7. Pang, Z.; Raudonis, R.; Glick, B.R.; Lina, T.J.; Cheng, Z. Antibiotic resistance in Pseudomonas aeruginosa: Mechanisms and alternative therapeutic strategies. *Biotechnol. Adv.* **2019**, *37*, 177–192. [CrossRef] [PubMed]
8. Mulcahy, L.R.; Jane, L.B.; Stephen, L.; Kim, L. Emergence of Pseudomonas aeruginosa strains producing high levels of persister cells in patients with cystic fibrosis. *J. Bacteriol. Res.* **2010**, *192*, 6191–6199. [CrossRef] [PubMed]
9. Breidenstein, E.B.; Elena, B.M.; de la Fuente-Núñez, C.; Robert, E.H. Pseudomonas aeruginosa: All roads lead to resistance. *Trends Microbiol.* **2011**, *19*, 419–426. [CrossRef] [PubMed]
10. Blair, J.M.; Vassiliy, N.B.; Vito, R.; Niraj, M.; Pierpaolo, C.; Ulrich, K.; Paolo, R.; Vargiu, A.; Baylay, A.; Smith, H.; et al. AcrB drug-binding pocket substitution confers clinically relevant resistance and altered substrate specificity. *Proc. Natl. Acad. Sci. USA* **2015**, *112*, 3511–3516. [CrossRef] [PubMed]
11. Suresh, M.; Narayanan, N.; Vimal, K.; Jayasree, P.; Kumar, P. Mutational and Phylogenetic Analysis of nfxB Gene in Multidrug-Resistant Clinical Isolates of Pseudomonas aeruginosa Hyperexpressing MexCD-OprJ Efflux Pump. *Adv. Microbiol.* **2019**, *9*, 993. [CrossRef]
12. Kohler, T.; Michéa-Hamzehpour, M.; Henze, U.; Gotoh, N.; Kocjancic, C.L.; Pechère, J. Characterization of MexE–MexF–OprN, a positively regulated multidrug efflux system of Pseudomonas aeruginosa. *Mol. Microbiol.* **1997**, *23*, 345–354. [CrossRef] [PubMed]
13. Bialvaei, A.Z.; Rahbar, M.; Hamidi-Farahani, R.; Asgari, A.; Esmailkhani, A.; Soleiman-Meigooni, S. Expression of RND efflux pumps mediated antibiotic resistance in Pseudomonas aeruginosa clinical strains. *Microb. Pathog.* **2021**, *153*, 104789. [CrossRef] [PubMed]
14. Younes, K.; Memar, M.Y.; Farajnia, S.; Adibkia, K.; Kafil, H.S.; Ghotaslou, R. Molecular epidemiology and carbapenem resistance of Pseudomonas aeruginosa isolated from patients with burns. *J. Wound Care* **2021**, *30*, 2.
15. Mohseni, N.; Rad, M.; Khorramian Toosi, B.; Mokhtari, A.R.; Yahyaraeyat, R.; Salehi, T.Z. Evaluation of MexAB-OprM efflux pump and determination of antimicrobial susceptibility in Pseudomonas aeruginosa human and veterinary isolates. *Bulg. J. Vet. Med.* **2019**, *24*, 200–207. [CrossRef]
16. Ehiagbe, I.; Ehiagbe, F.; Akinshipe, B.; Ilobanafor, R. Fluoroquinolone efflux pump of Pseudomonas aeruginosa. *NISEB J.* **2019**, *11*, 4.
17. Rudy, M.A.; Dolatabadi, S.; Zare, H.; Ghazvini, K. Characterization of efflux pump-mediated resistance against fluoro-quinolones among clinical isolates of Pseudomonas aeruginosa in the northeast of Iran and its association with mortality of infected patients. *Cell* **2019**, *98*, 1248938.
18. Ali, Z.; Mumtaz, N.; Naz, S.A.; Jabeen, N.; Shafique, M. Multi-Drug Resistant Pseudomonas Aeruginosa: A threat of nosocomial infections in tertiary care hospitals. *J. Pak. Med. Assoc.* **2015**, *65*, 12. [PubMed]
19. Kishk, R.; Abdalla, M.; Hashish, A.; Nemr, N.; El Nahhas, N.; Alkahtani, S.; Abdel-Daim, M.; Kishk, S. Efflux MexAB-mediated resistance in P. aeruginosa isolated from patients with healthcare associated infections. *Pathogens* **2020**, *9*, 471. [CrossRef] [PubMed]

antibiotics

MDPI

Article

In Vitro Synergistic Activity of Antimicrobial Combinations against Carbapenem- and Colistin-Resistant *Acinetobacter baumannii* and *Klebsiella pneumoniae*

Paraskevi Mantzana, Efthymia Protonotariou, Angeliki Kassomenaki, Georgios Meletis *, Areti Tychala , Eirini Keskilidou, Maria Arhonti, Charikleia Katsanou, Aikaterini Daviti, Olga Vasilaki, Georgia Kagkalou and Lemonia Skoura

Department of Microbiology, School of Medicine, AHEPA University Hospital, Aristotle University of Thessaloniki, S. Kiriakidi str. 1, 54636 Thessaloniki, Greece

* Correspondence: meletisg@hotmail.com; Tel.: +30-6974282575

Abstract: Polymyxins are commonly used as the last resort for the treatment of MDR *Acinetobacter baumannii* and *Klebsiella pneumoniae* nosocomial infections; however, apart from the already known toxicity issues, resistance to these agents is emerging. In the present study, we assessed the in vitro synergistic activity of antimicrobial combinations against carbapenem-resistant and colistin-resistant *A. baumannii* and *K. pneumoniae* in an effort to provide more options for their treatment. Two hundred *A. baumannii* and one hundred and six *K. pneumoniae* single clinical isolates with resistance to carbapenems and colistin, recovered between 1 January 2021 and 31 July 2022,were included. *A. baumannii* were tested by the MIC test strip fixed-ratio method for combinations of colistin with either meropenem or rifampicin or daptomycin. *K. pneumoniae* were tested for the combinations of colistin with meropenem and ceftazidime/avibactam with aztreonam. Synergy was observed at: 98.99% for colistin and meropenem against *A. baumannii*; 91.52% for colistin and rifampicin; and 100% for colistin and daptomycin. Synergy was also observed at: 73.56% for colistin and meropenem against *K. pneumoniae* and; and 93% for ceftazidime/avibactam with aztreonam. The tested antimicrobial combinations presented high synergy rates, rendering them valuable options against *A. baumannii* and *K. pneumoniae* infections.

Keywords: synergistic activity; colistin; meropenem; imipenem; ceftazidime/avibactam; rifampicin; daptomycin; fosfomycin; aztreonam; amikacin

1. Introduction

Infections caused by antimicrobial-resistant Gram-negative pathogens are a healthcare issue of major importance and are associated with poor patient outcomes [1,2]. *Acinetobacter baumannii* and *Klebsiella pneumoniae* often develop mechanisms to evade the action of antimicrobials and can acquire genes encoding for antimicrobial resistance mechanisms. Among them, carbapenemases are the most clinically important [3]. The extent of resistance of each isolate may vary; therefore, different definitions may be applied: multi-drug resistant (MDR) refers to an isolate that is resistant to three or more antimicrobial categories, extensively drug resistant (XDR) refers to an isolate that is susceptible to only one last resort antimicrobial and pan-drug resistant (PDR) refers to an isolate that is resistant to all available antimicrobials [4].

The presence and spread of MDR, XDR and even PDR Gram-negatives is dramatically limiting the treatment options for infections caused by these pathogens, whereas the pipeline of new antimicrobials is slow and novel compounds including tigecycline, eravacycline and cefiderocol do not always meet the expectations [5–7]. Current β-lactams combined with novel β-lactamase inhibitors provide some solutions especially against non-metallo-β-lactamase producers [8], but they are not applicable in all cases, and resistance has already emerged [9,10]. Monotherapy with formerly abandoned antimicrobials such as fosfomycin and polymyxins is another option. However, it presents limitations including dosing issues for fosfomycin [11], nephrotoxicity for polymyxins [12] and resistance development for both [13,14].

The combined use of two antimicrobial agents has been used in the management of infectious diseases for decades, garnering more attention lately due to the aforementioned reasons. Combined treatment may prevent resistance selection, reduce dose-related toxicity as a result of reduced dosage of a specific compound, but more importantly in the case of MDR Gram-negatives, it is expected to provide a probable synergy between the two antimicrobials. On the other hand, potential disadvantages may include the increased cost, a greater risk for combined toxicity and the development of even more resistant bacteria [15]. Clinicians are increasingly prescribing combination therapy for the treatment of carbapenem-resistant Gram-negative bacteria according to a recent survey in large hospitals in Europe and the United States [16]. However, they are often driven empirically to the selection of the combined antimicrobials based on trial which may lead to inadequate patient care. A recent meta-analysis showed that synergy-guided antimicrobial combination therapy against MDR-GNB was significantly associated with survival [17].

Over the past years, *A. baumanni* and *K. pneumoniae* have emerged as serious nosocomial pathogens especially due to their extensively resistant antimicrobial profile [18]. Polymyxin (colistin or polymyxin B) is currently used as one of the last resort agents to treat the related infections, but resistance because of monotherapy urges the need to find effective antimicrobial combinations to overcome this problem. The combinations used most commonly include a polymyxin together with a carbapenem [16]. In the present study, we retrospectively evaluated the in vitro effectiveness of selected antimicrobial combinations against carbapenem- and colistin-resistant *A. baumannii* and *K. pneumoniae* clinical isolates.

2. Results

2.1. *Acinetobacter baumannii*

The studied isolates displayed high rates of resistance to major classes of antimicrobials with 100% resistance to carbapenems and colistin (Table 1). The MIC_{50} and MIC_{90} for tigecycline were 3 mg/L and 6 mg/L; for ampicillin/sulbactam, ≥32 mg/L and ≥32 mg/L; for rifampicin, 6 mg/L and 32 mg/L; and for daptomycin, ≥256 mg/L and ≥256 mg/L, respectively. One hundred and ninety-eight isolates were tested for the colistin–meropenem combination exhibiting 98.99% (196/198) synergy (FICI range = 0.001–0.5) and 1.01% (2/198) additivity (FICI = 0.563). Although rifampicin and daptomycin are typically inactive against Gram-negative bacteria, high synergy rates were observed using the colistin–rifampicin combination with 91.52% (162/177) synergy (FICI range = 0.002–0.5); 7.91% (14/177) additivity (FICI range = 0.52–0.917) and 0.57% (1/177) indifference (FICI = 1.125). The colistin–daptomycin combination was tested in 129 isolates, resulting in 100% synergy (FICI range = 0.002–0.5) (Supplementary Table S1 and Figure 1).

Table 1. Antimicrobial profile of *A. baumannii* isolates. NA: not applicable.

Antimicrobial	Number of Isolates Tested	MIC Range (mg/L)	MIC_{50} (mg/L)	MIC_{90} (mg/L)	Resistance (%)
Meropenem	200	8–≥16	≥16	≥16	100
Imipenem	200	≥16	≥16	≥16	100
Colistin	200	4–≥16	≥16	≥16	100
Ciprofloxacin	200	≥4	≥4	≥4	100
Amikacin	136	4–≥64	≥64	≥64	97.79
Gentamicin	133	1–≥16	≥16	≥16	98.49
Ampicillin/Sulbactam	158	16–≥32	≥32	≥32	NA
Tigecycline	192	0.047–12	3	6	NA
Rifampicin	178	1–≥256	6	32	NA
Daptomycin	128	≥256	≥256	≥256	NA

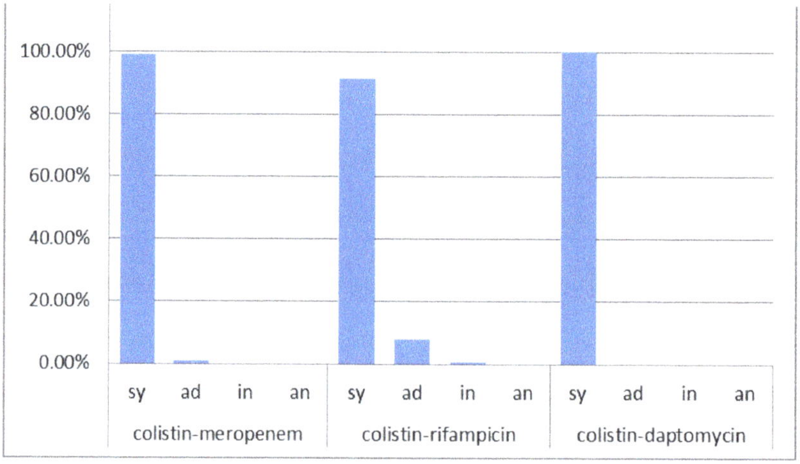

Figure 1. The% results of antimicrobial combinations tested for *A. baumannii*. sy: synergy; ad: additivity; in: indifference; an: antagonism.

2.2. *Klebsiella pneumoniae*

The *K. pneumoniae* isolates presented 100% resistance to carbapenems and colistin (Table 2). The resistance rate to ceftazidime/avibactam was 87.50% (the MIC_{50} and MIC_{90} were both ≥16 mg/L). Sixty-four were metallo-β-lactamase (MBL) producers, 13 were *Klebsiella pneumoniae* carbapenemase (KPC) producers and 29 were positive for both carbapenemase types. Eighty-seven isolates were tested for the colistin–meropenem combination exhibiting 73.56% (64/87) synergy (FICI range = 0.014–0.5); 13.80% (12/87) additivity (FICI range = 0.75–0.938); and 12.64% (11/87) indifference (FICI range = 1–2). Specifically, synergy rates of 66.7% (34/51), 90.9% (10/13) and 80% (20/25) were observed for MBL, KPC and MBL+KPC strains, respectively. For the ceftazidime/avibactam combination with aztreonam, the following were shown: 93% (93/100) synergy (FICI range = 0.0007–0.5); 3% (3/100) additivity (FICI range = 0.625–0.938); and 4% (4/100) indifference (FICI range = 1.25–4); no antagonism was observed (Supplementary Table S2 and Figure 2). Of the 62 MBL strains tested for the combination ceftazidime/avibactam with aztreonam, 95.2% (59/62) exhibited synergy, 3.2% (2/62) exhibited additivity and 1.6% (1/62) showed indifference, while all (10/10) of KPC-producing strains showed synergy. Lower rates of synergy, i.e., 85.7% (24/28), were observed for the strains with both carbapenemase types.

Table 2. Antimicrobial profile of *K. pneumoniae* isolates. NA: not applicable.

Antimicrobial	Number of Isolates Tested	MIC Range (mg/L)	MIC_{50} (mg/L)	MIC_{90} (mg/L)	Resistance (%)
Meropenem	106	≥16	≥16	≥16	100
Imipenem	106	≥16	≥16	≥16	100
Colistin	106	4–≥16	≥16	≥16	100
Ceftazidime/Avibactam	104	1–≥16	≥16	≥16	87.50
Ceftazidime	103	16–≥64	≥64	≥64	100
Ceftolozane/Tazobactam	83	≥32	≥32	≥32	100
Cefotaxime	81	2–≥64	≥64	≥64	96.29
Aztreonam	104	16–≥64	≥64	≥64	100
Ciprofloxacin	102	0.25–≥4	≥4	≥4	99.01
Amikacin	104	2–≥64	32	≥64	97.11
Gentamicin	101	1–≥16	≥16	≥16	93.06
Piperacillin/Tazobactam	102	≥128	≥128	≥128	100
Fosfomycin	102	16–≥256	256	≥256	90.19
Tigecycline	92	0.25–8	2	8	NA
Chloramphenicol	91	2–≥64	32	≥64	87.91

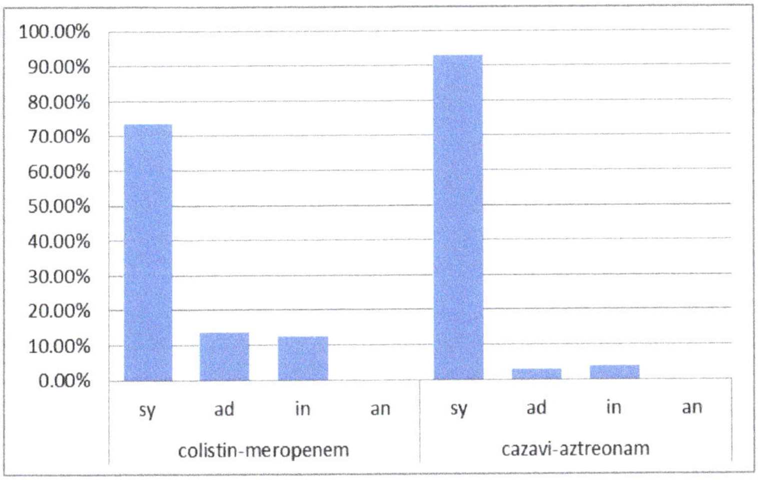

Figure 2. The % results of antimicrobial combinations tested for *K. pneumoniae*. cazavi: ceftazidime/avibactam; sy: synergy; ad: additivity; in: indifference; an: antagonism.

3. Discussion

According to the most recent epidemiological data from the Antimicrobial resistance Surveillance report in Europe, 21 countries, mostly in southern and eastern Europe, showed rates of *Acinetobacter* resistance to carbapenems equal to or above 50%, with 96.9% for Greece (https://www.ecdc.europa.eu/sites/default/files/documents/Surveillance-antimicrobial-resistance-in-Europe-2020.pdf) (accessed on 1 December 2022). This poses a great public health threat to patients and healthcare systems, with an estimated 2363 attributable deaths in 2015 in countries of the European Union (EU)/European Economic Area (EEA) [19]. Almost a quarter of EU/EEA countries reported carbapenem resistance percentages above 10% in *K. pneumonia*, while Greece had a rate of 73.7%.

Polymyxin, in some cases, is the only resort agent for the treatment of MDR and XDR Gram-negatives, but efficacy may be suboptimal in several infections according to the pharmacokinetic (PK) and pharmacodynamic (PD) data, even with the highest tolerable therapeutic dose [20]. Monotherapy may lead to resistance as well, probably due to the selection of pre-existing colistin-resistant subpopulations in heteroresistant strains [21] or emergence of chromosomal mutations besides the transmission of plasmid-mediated resistance [15,22–24]. Increased rates of colistin resistance have been reported all over the world, especially in Eastern Mediterranean countries and South East Asia, with a rate of 4% for Greece in the period2012–2016 [25]. Resistance to colistin was 47.7% among *A. baumannii* isolates from patients with ventilator-associated pneumonia in Greece, Italy and Spain [26]. According to a recent meta-analysis by Karakonstantis et al., the pooled rate of *A. baumannii* colistin heteroresistance was 33% [24]. Specifically for *K. pneumoniae* isolated from bloodstream infections, the pooled rate of resistance was increased to 12.90% for studies in 2020 and beyond, compared to 2.89% in the period 2015–2019 [27].

Combination regimens with colistin have been proposed to overcome the re-growth after colistin monotherapy either by reducing resistance or by enhancing bacterial killing through synergy between the two antimicrobials. Better antimicrobial effect is achieved by sub-population or mechanistic synergy that can act concomitantly. Sub-population synergy is a process where the resistant sub-populations of one antimicrobial are killed by the other and the opposite. Mechanistic synergy refers to two antimicrobials with different mode of action that enhance the killing of one another. Colistin, for example, seems to increase the permeability of the outer membrane of Gram-negatives.

It should be pointed out that methods for synergy testing are not completely standardized, and there are variations concerning the interpretation of synergy [28]. Most studies use time-kill assays and checkerboard as these are considered standard methods for antimicrobial combinations testing [28,29]. These are, however, time-consuming and laborious for a clinical microbiology laboratory. Gradient diffusion methods are widely used and easy to perform and, thus, can be more easily integrated in a routine base for synergy testing [28]. Since our laboratory is a clinical diagnostic lab, we chose the MIC gradient synergy testing due to the increased daily workload. For synergy interpretation, we used the most recent criteria of antagonism defined as FICI > 4 [15].

Antimicrobials selected for synergy in our study were bactericidal, since a recent meta-analysis showed that combinations including bactericidal antimicrobials had better synergy rates, while most antagonistic effects were demonstrated when a bacteriostatic antimicrobial was included [28].

Recently published studies demonstrated in vitro synergistic effect for the combinations of polymyxin with a carbapenem, rifampicin or a glycopeptide for colistin-susceptible but also colistin-resistant MDR or XDR *A. baumannii* isolates [30]. On the contrary, multiple studies testing colistin paired with tigecycline failed to achieve synergy in vitro and in vivo compared with polymyxin/carbapenem combinations [31] and resulted in a lesser microbiological cure [32]. A systematic review and meta-analysis that included only killing assay (PK/PD and time-killing) studies showed high level of synergy for polymyxin/meropenem and polymyxin-rifampicin combinations against *A. baumannii* isolates [33].

The combinations used most include a polymyxin together with a carbapenem. Systematic reviews and meta-analysis with *A. baumannii* strains showed pooled synergy rates of 17.5–98.3% for polymyxin-carbapenem combinations [34–36]. The great fluctuation is depending on the different applied method for synergy, with higher rates reported for time-kill assays but also on the number of isolates tested, their different susceptibility profile and the clonal diversity of strains [36,37]. The synergy rate for meropenem was higher than that of imipenem (85.2–86% vs. 56–66.2%, respectively). For polymyxin-resistant strains, the synergy rate was above 50% [34,36]. Our study exhibited a high rate 98.99% of synergy for *A. baumannii* strains against the combination of colistin–meropenem, similarly to the 96% rate of a recent study with colistin-resistant strains [38]. A study that compared colistin–meropenem against colistin-resistant (CoR) and colistin-susceptible (CoS) *A. baumannii* isolates showed increased rates of synergy for the CoR group (85.4% vs. 4.9% for the CoS group) [39]. Low rates of antagonism were observed in previous studies [36], whereas none of our strains exhibited antagonism.

Recent studies pointed out the paradoxical phenomenon of CoR Gram-negatives strains showing increased susceptibility to drugs usually inactive against Gram-negatives such as rifampicin, daptomycin, glycopeptides or macrolides [15]. A possible explanation might be the increased permeability due to the alteration of the outer membrane which allows the entrance of those drugs. Data from systematic reviews and meta-analyses showed high rates of synergy for the pair polymyxin-rifampicin [30,33,34] and specifically for CoR strains 56.8%, similarlyto CoS. Three randomized controlled trials showed that colistin–rifampicin managed an increased rate of microbiological eradication but had no effect on mortality or length of hospitalization [40–42]. A study with CoR *A. baumannii* strains exhibited higher synergy rates than CoS for the colistin–rifampicin pair (80.5% vs. 14.6% respectively) [39]. This is in accordance with the high rate of synergy 91.52% observed in our CoR strains. Decreased values of MICs of rifampicin alone were observed in our study (MIC_5), similarly to one study with CoR strains [43].

Colistin combined with daptomycin has proved very efficient against our CoR *A. baumannii* strains with 100% synergy. On the contrary, a study evaluating this combination against XDR *Acinetobacter* strains with time-kill assays showed synergistic effect only against CoS and indifference against CoR, but the different synergy methodology must be taken into account [44]. Few studies have evaluated this combination; however, no antagonism was observed [44–46]. To the best of our knowledge, our collection is the largest evaluating the colistin–daptomycin combination.

The most prevalent mechanism of resistance for *K. pneumoniae* is the production of β-lactamases with a geographical distribution [47]. The novel β-lactam/β-lactamase inhibitor combinations are used against non-metallo-β-lactamase-producing strains, but for MBL-producers, the treatment choices are limited. Many studies have proposed the combination of ceftazidime/avibactam plus aztreonam for MBL strains with high synergy rates [48–53]. As aztreonam is not hydrolyzed by MBLs, the addition of avibactam can inhibit other β-lactamases (ESBLs, AmpCs, serine carbapenemases) if present and thus restore the susceptibility to aztreonam [49,54]. In our study, 87.65% showed synergy to this combination in accordance with a study including only CoR carbapenem-resistant isolates [55]. Specifically for MBL-producing strains a rate of 95.2% was observed, while strains with both carbapenemase types had a lower rate of 85.7%. As expected, the combination exhibited synergistic effect for the small number of KPC isolates tested as they are already susceptible to ceftazidime/avibactam. An observational prospective study in patients with bloodstream infections caused by MBL-producing Enterobacterales, mainly *K. pneumoniae*, showed better clinical response for the ceftazidime/avibactam plus aztreonam combination than other therapeutic agents [56]. The Infectious Diseases Society of America (IDSA) recommends this combination for the treatment of MBL-producing CRE (https://www.idsociety.org/practice-guideline/amr-guidance/) (accessed on 1 December 2022), while the aztreonam/avibactam drug combination is pending a phase III clinical trial (https://www.clinicaltrialsregister.eu/ctr-search/search?query=aztreonam-avibactam) (accessed on 1 December 2022). Meanwhile, many studies have proved the efficacy of aztreonam/avibactam for the treatment of CRE, including MBLproduction [57–59].

The pooled synergy rate for the combination of colistin–carbapenem against *K. pneumoniae* was 44% in a meta-analysis, and when examining CoR *K. pneumoniae* isolates, the rate increased to 62% [36]. A synergy rate of 73.56% for the combination of colistin plus meropenem was observed in our study. Although KPC is the predominant mechanism of resistance for *K. pneumoniae* strains in our hospital (data not shown) we only included 13 KPC strains, as ceftazidime/avibactam can be used as a therapy for these isolates. This drug, however, may not be available in every hospital; thus, alternative therapeutic options must be taken into account. With a synergy rate of 90.9% in our study, colistin–meropenem could be used in the absence of ceftazidime/avibactam. Lower rates were observed for MBL (66.7%, 34/51) and MBL+KPC strains (80%, 20/25), indicating that the combination of ceftazidime/avibactam plus aztreonam is more synergistic than colistin–meropenem.

Randomized controlled trials failed to show reduction in all-over mortality in the group of patients receiving combination therapy compared to colistin monotherapy [40–42,60]. A multinational observational retrospective study among patients with CRE bloodstream infections (INCREMENT) demonstrated that combination therapy was associated with lower mortality than monotherapy only in patients with a high mortality score [61]. On the other hand, colistin combinations with carbapenems, rifampicin and sulbactam were related to a higher microbiological effect compared to colistin monotherapy against *A. baumannii* strains [32,62]. This may be due to the fact that microbiological response represents the effect of the drug, but other factors might be responsible for the clinical deterioration [32]. Interestingly, a lower mortality rate was observed in the subgroup of CoR *Acinetobacter* strains of the AIDA study for colistin–meropenem combination compared to colistin monotherapy [63]. Resistance to colistin usually contributes to fitness cost, and the administration of meropenem may restore virulence through gene expression changes. Unfortunately, data on synergy were not reported on this subgroup [63]. This would be significant, as the results of combination synergy against particular isolates does not reflect all *Acinetobacter* strains [64]. Further studies are needed to support this result. Discrepancy between in vitro testing and clinical trial results may be due to the pharmacokinetics of colistin with a great variability especially among critically ill patients, the concomitant co-morbidities, the specific pathogen and resistance mechanism, the site of infection (the respiratory tract is not easily accessible either for colistin or other antimicrobials) and the delay on the administration of empirical treatment [15,65].

Our study presents some limitations. First of all, our results refer to the in vitro activity of the studied antimicrobial combinations and should be interpreted in the context that in vitro susceptibility data are not the only parameter that has to be taken into account when deciding the proper antimicrobial treatment for each patient. Clinical management is a dynamic process with individualized adjustment chemotherapy over time. Second, even though we included only single-patient isolates, we were not able to employ sequencing-based methods to better characterize the molecular epidemiology of the strains implemented in our study. Third, it is well known that diffusion methods are generally not recommended for colistin, because its large molecule does not diffuse as much as other antimicrobials in agar plates. However, the MIC test strip fixed-ratio method is acceptably labor intensive for clinical laboratories and is used for the in vitro synergistic activity testing of antimicrobial combinations including colistin [39]. Finally, our work is a single-center study and does not necessarily reflect the whole picture regarding the susceptibility of strains isolated in other institutions. Therefore, we strongly recommend the antimicrobial combination testing for each XDR or PDR isolate, especially in cases presenting resistance to polymyxins.

4. Materials and Methods

4.1. Study Design

Two hundred *A. baumannii* single clinical isolates with resistance to carbapenems and colistin between 1 January 2021 and 31 July 2022 were included in the study; 81 were isolated from blood, 76 from bronchoalveolar secretions, 21 from urine, 7 from sputum, 6 from central lines, 4 from wound cultures, 3 from biopsy and soft tissues, and 1 from pus, pleural fluid and cerebrospinal fluid, respectively. A total of 198 isolates were tested for colistin and meropenem synergy; 177 were tested for the colistin and rifampicin combination; and 129 were tested for colistin and daptomycin.

A total of 106 *K. pneumoniae* single clinical isolates with resistance to carbapenems and colistin were also included; 32 were isolated from bronchoalveolar secretions, 31 from urine, 30 from blood, 8 from central line catheters, 4 from wound infections and 1 from sputum. Overall, 87 were tested for colistin and meropenem synergy and 100 for the ceftazidime/avibactam plus aztreonam combination.

Antimicrobial susceptibility testing was performed by the Vitek2 (bioMérieux, Marcy-l'Étoile, France), where applicable. Tigecycline, rifampicin and daptomycin were tested with MIC test strips (Liofilchem, Roseto degli Abruzzi, Teramo, Italy). Colistin susceptibility was performed by the broth microdilution method (Liofilchem, Roseto degli Abruzzi, Teramo, Italy). MIC ranges, MIC_{50} and MIC_{90} were calculated for the antimicrobials tested. Antimicrobial resistance rates were calculated according to the EUCAST breakpoints v 12.0 (2022). In vitro synergistic activity testing of antimicrobial combinations was performed using the MIC test strip fixed-ratio method.

4.2. MIC Test Strip Fixed-Ratio Method

The MIC test strip fixed-ratio method [37] was used for the synergistic activity of antimicrobial combinations using MIC test strips of both antimicrobials for each antimicrobial combination. Three antimicrobial combinations of colistin with either meropenem or rifampicin or daptomycin were tested for *A. baumannii*. Colistin with meropenem and ceftazidime/avibactam with aztreonam were tested for *K. pneumoniae*. Briefly, a 0.5 McFarland solution was prepared and inoculated onto a Mueller Hinton agar plate. The MIC strip of the first antimicrobial (antimicrobial agent A) was placed and left for 1 h, at room temperature, to allow the antimicrobial to diffuse into the medium. Afterwards, the MIC strip of antimicrobial A was removed, cleaned with alcohol and saved as MIC template reading scale. The MIC strip of the second antimicrobial (antimicrobial agent B) was then placed directly over the imprint of A with the highest concentrations coinciding. In parallel, plates with an MIC strip of each antimicrobial alone were prepared. The plates were incubated, at 36–37 °C, for 18–24 h, and the MICs of each drug alone along with the MIC of the drugs in combination were assessed with the use of the respective MIC strip/scales. The results were interpreted using the fractional inhibitory concentration index (FICI) [66] calculated as:

$$FICI = FIC_{agentA} + FIC_{agentB} = MIC_{AB}/MIC_A + MIC_{BA}/MIC_B \quad (1)$$

MIC_{AB} is the MIC of A in the presence of B; MIC_{BA} is the MIC of B in the presence of A; MIC_A and MIC_B are the MICs of each drug alone. 'Synergy', 'additivity', 'indifference' and 'antagonism' were interpreted when the FICI was $\leq$0.5, >0.5–$\leq$1, >1–$\leq$4 and >4, respectively. Synergy is considered the interaction of the two antimicrobials to increase each other's effect; additivity means the additional effect of the action of two antimicrobials without synergism; antagonism suggests that the combined effect of the two antimicrobials is less than the most effective one used individually; and indifference indicates the absence of all the aforementioned phenomena.

4.3. *Phenotypic Detection of* K. pneumoniae *Carbapenem Resistance Mechanisms*

For the phenotypic detection of MBL or KPC production, the double meropenem disc test was used. The double meropenem disc test is a combined disc test using meropenem discs with and without the carbapenemase inhibitors EDTA and phenylboronic acid. Briefly, a 0.5 McFarland bacterial suspension was prepared and inoculated onto a Mueller Hinton agar plate. Four meropenem discs were placed on the surface of the agar. One was left without inhibitors. On the second disc, 10 μL of EDTA 0.1 M was added. Phenylboronic acid (20 g/L) was added on the third disc. Finally, both inhibitors were added on the fourth disc. After 18–24 h of incubation, the evaluation of the result was performed as follows: The absence of inhibition zone around the first disc or an inhibition zone of <22 mm indicated carbapenem resistance. The presence of an inhibition zone around the second and the fourth disc with a diameter $\geq$5 mm wider than that of the first disc was indicative of MBL production. The presence of an inhibition zone around the third and the fourth disc with a diameter $\geq$5 mm wider than that of the first disc was indicative of KPC production. The presence of an inhibition zone around the second and third disc with a diameter $\geq$5 mm wider than that of the first disc and an even larger inhibition zone around the fourth disc was indicative of both MBL and KPC production.

5. Conclusions

In vitro colistin-based combinations with either meropenem or rifampicin or daptomycin resulted in high synergy rates, rendering them a valuable option for the treatment of colistin-resistant *A. baumannii* infections. The same applies for ceftazidime/avibactam-aztreonam and colistin–meropenem combinations against difficult to treat *K. pneumoniae* infections. MIC gradient synergy testing can serve as a simple tool in clinical microbiological laboratories guiding clinicians to the proper therapy for these resistant pathogens.

Supplementary Materials: The following supporting information can be downloaded at: https://www.mdpi.com/article/10.3390/antibiotics12010093/s1, Table S1: Results of antimicrobial combinations tested for *A. baumannii*; Table S2: Results of antimicrobial combinations tested for *K. pneumoniae*.

Author Contributions: P.M. contributed to conception, supervision and design, and drafted the manuscript. E.P. contributed to conception, supervision and design, and drafted the manuscript. A.K. contributed to data acquisition and interpretation and drafted the manuscript. G.M. contributed to design, data acquisition and data interpretation, and drafted the manuscript. A.T. contributed to data acquisition and interpretation. E.K. contributed to data acquisition. M.A. contributed to data acquisition. C.K. contributed to data acquisition. A.D. contributed to data acquisition. O.V. contributed to data acquisition and interpretation. G.K. to data acquisition and contributed to data acquisition and interpretation. L.S. contributed to supervision and interpretation, and critically revised the manuscript. All authors have read and agreed to the published version of the manuscript.

Funding: This research received no external funding.

Institutional Review Board Statement: Not applicable.

Informed Consent Statement: Not applicable.

Data Availability Statement: Not applicable.

Conflicts of Interest: The authors declare no conflict of interest. Part of this study was presentedas a poster at the 2nd International Electronic Conference on antimicrobials—Drugs for Superbugs: antimicrobial Discovery, Modes of Action and Mechanisms of Resistance.

References

1. Vardakas, K.Z.; Rafailidis, P.I.; Konstantelias, A.A.; Falagas, M.E. Predictors of mortality in patients with infections due to multi-drug resistant Gram negative bacteria: The study, the patient, the bug or the drug? *J. Infect.* **2013**, *66*, 401–414. [CrossRef] [PubMed]
2. Lemos, E.V.; de la Hoz, F.P.; Alvis, N.; Einarson, T.R.; Quevedo, E.; Castañeda, C.; Leon, Y.; Amado, C.; Cañon, O.; Kawai, K. Impact of carbapenem resistance on clinical and economic outcomes among patients with *Acinetobacter baumannii* infection in Colombia. *Clin. Microbiol. Infect.* **2014**, *20*, 174–180. [CrossRef] [PubMed]
3. Meletis, G. Carbapenem resistance: Overview of the problem and future perspectives. *Ther. Adv. Infect. Dis.* **2016**, *3*, 15–21. [CrossRef] [PubMed]
4. Magiorakos, A.P.; Srinivasan, A.; Carey, R.B.; Carmeli, Y.; Falagas, M.E.; Giske, C.G.; Harbarth, S.; Hindler, J.F.; Kahlmeter, G.; Olsson-Liljequist, B.; et al. Multidrug-resistant, extensively drug-resistant and pandrug-resistant bacteria: An international expert proposal for interim standard definitions for acquired resistance. *Clin. Microbiol. Infect.* **2012**, *18*, 268–281. [CrossRef]
5. Seifert, H.; Blondeau, J.; Lucaßen, K.; Utt, E.A. Global update on the in vitro activity of tigecycline and comparators against isolates of *Acinetobacter baumannii* and rates of resistant phenotypes (2016–2018). *J. Glob. Antimicrob. Resist.* **2022**, *31*, 82–89. [CrossRef]
6. Meletis, G.; Protonotariou, E.; Gkeka, I.; Kassomenaki, A.; Mantzana, P.; Tychala, A.; Vlachodimou, N.; Kourti, A.; Skoura, L. In vitro activity of eravacycline and cefoperazone/sulbactam against extensively-drug resistant and pan-drug resistant *Acinetobacter baumannii* isolates from a tertiary hospital in Greece. *New Microbiol.* **2022**, *45*, 210–212.
7. Smoke, S.M.; Brophy, A.; Reveron, S.; Iovleva, A.; Kline, E.G.; Marano, M.; Miller, L.P.; Shields, R.K. Evolution and transmission of cefiderocol-resistant *Acinetobacter baumannii* during an outbreak in the burn intensive care unit. *Clin. Infect. Dis.* **2022**, ciac647. [CrossRef]
8. Zhen, S.; Wang, H.; Feng, S. Update of clinical application in ceftazidime-avibactam for multidrug-resistant Gram-negative bacteria infections. *Infection* **2022**, *50*, 1409–1423. [CrossRef]
9. Xiong, L.; Wang, X.; Wang, Y.; Yu, W.; Zhou, Y.; Chi, X.; Xiao, T.; Xiao, Y. Molecular mechanisms underlying bacterial resistance to ceftazidime/avibactam. *WIREs Mech. Dis.* **2022**, *14*, e1571. [CrossRef]
10. Jiang, M.; Sun, B.; Huang, Y.; Liu, C.; Wang, Y.; Ren, Y.; Zhang, Y.; Wang, Y.; Mu, D. Diversity of ceftazidime-avibactam resistance mechanism in KPC2-producing *Klebsiella pneumoniae* under antimicrobial selection pressure. *Infect. Drug Resist.* **2022**, *15*, 4627–4636. [CrossRef]
11. Williams, P.C. Potential of fosfomycin in treating multidrug-resistant infections in children. *J. Paediatr. Child Health* **2020**, *56*, 864–872. [CrossRef] [PubMed]
12. Jafari, F.; Elyasi, S. Prevention of colistin induced nephrotoxicity: A review of preclinical and clinical data. *Expert Rev. Clin. Pharmacol.* **2021**, *14*, 1113–1131. [CrossRef] [PubMed]
13. Ríos, E.; Del Carmen López Diaz, M.; Culebras, E.; Rodríguez-Avial, I.; Rodríguez-Avial, C. Resistance to fosfomycin is increasing and is significantly associated with extended-spectrum β-lactamase-production in urinary isolates of *Escherichia coli*. *Med. Microbiol. Immunol.* **2022**, *211*, 269–272. [CrossRef]
14. Meletis, G.; Skoura, L. Polymyxin resistance mechanisms: From intrinsic resistance to mcr genes. *Recent Pat. Antiinfect. Drug Discov.* **2018**, *13*, 198–206. [CrossRef] [PubMed]
15. Bergen, P.J.; Smith, N.M.; Bedard, T.B.; Bulman, Z.P.; Cha, R.; Tsuji, B.T. Rational combinations of polymyxins with other antibiotics. *Adv. Exp. Med. Biol.* **2019**, *1145*, 251–288. [PubMed]
16. Papst, L.; Beović, B.; Pulcini, C.; Durante-Mangoni, E.; Rodríguez-Baño, J.; Kaye, K.S.; Daikos, G.L.; Raka, L.; Paul, M.; ESGAP, ESGBIS, ESGIE and the CRGNB treatment survey study group. Antibiotic treatment of infections caused by carbapenem-resistant Gram-negative bacilli: An international ESCMID cross-sectional survey among infectious diseases specialists practicing in large hospitals. *Clin. Microbiol. Infect.* **2018**, *24*, 1070–1076. [CrossRef]
17. Vardakas, K.Z.; Athanassaki, F.; Pitiriga, V.; Falagas, M.E. Clinical relevance of in vitro synergistic activity of antibiotics for multidrug-resistant Gram-negative infections: A systematic review. *J. Glob. Antimicrob. Resist.* **2019**, *17*, 250–259. [CrossRef]
18. Mancuso, G.; Midiri, A.; Gerace, E.; Biondo, C. Bacterial antimicrobial resistance: The most critical pathogens. *Pathogens* **2021**, *10*, 1310. [CrossRef]

19. Cassini, A.; Högberg, L.D.; Plachouras, D.; Quattrocchi, A.; Hoxha, A.; Simonsen, G.S.; Colomb-Cotinat, M.; Kretzschmar, M.E.; Devleesschauwer, B.; Cecchini, M.; et al. Attributable deaths and disability-adjusted life-years caused by infections with antibiotic-resistant bacteria in the EU and the European Economic Area in 2015: A population-level modelling analysis. *Lancet Infect. Dis.* **2019**, *19*, 56–66. [CrossRef]
20. Piperaki, E.T.; Tzouvelekis, L.S.; Miriagou, V.; Daikos, G.L. Carbapenem-resistant *Acinetobacter baumannii*: In pursuit of an effective treatment. *Clin. Microbiol. Infect.* **2019**, *25*, 951–957. [CrossRef]
21. Meletis, G.; Tzampaz, E.; Sianou, E.; Tzavaras, I.; Sofianou, D. Colistin heteroresistance in carbapenemase-producing *Klebsiella pneumoniae*. *J. Antimicrob. Chemotherap.* **2011**, *66*, 946–947. [CrossRef] [PubMed]
22. El-Sayed Ahmed, M.A.E.; Zhong, L.L.; Shen, C.; Yang, Y.; Doi, Y.; Tian, G.B. Colistin and its role in the Era of antibiotic resistance: An extended review (2000–2019). *Emerg. Microbes Infect.* **2020**, *9*, 868–885. [CrossRef] [PubMed]
23. Karakonstantis, S.; Kritsotakis, E.I.; Gikas, A. Pandrug-resistant Gram-negative bacteria: A systematic review of current epidemiology, prognosis and treatment options. *J. Antimicrob. Chemother.* **2020**, *75*, 271–282. [CrossRef]
24. Karakonstantis, S.; Saridakis, I. Colistin heteroresistance in *Acinetobacter* spp.: Systematic review and meta-analysis of the prevalence and discussion of the mechanisms and potential therapeutic implications. *Int. J. Antimicrob. Agents* **2020**, *56*, 106065. [CrossRef] [PubMed]
25. Pormohammad, A.; Mehdinejadiani, K.; Gholizadeh, P.; Nasiri, M.J.; Mohtavinejad, N.; Dadashi, M.; Karimaei, S.; Safari, H.; Azimi, T. Global prevalence of colistin resistance in clinical isolates of *Acinetobacter baumannii*: A systematic review and meta-analysis. *Microb. Pathog.* **2020**, *139*, 103887. [CrossRef] [PubMed]
26. Nowak, J.; Zander, E.; Stefanik, D.; Higgins, P.G.; Roca, I.; Vila, J.; McConnell, M.J.; Cisneros, J.M.; Seifert, H.; MagicBullet Working Group WP4. High incidence of pandrug-resistant *Acinetobacter baumannii* isolates collected from patients with ventilator-associated pneumonia in Greece, Italy and Spain as part of the MagicBullet clinical trial. *J. Antimicrob. Chemother.* **2017**, *72*, 3277–3282. [CrossRef]
27. Uzairue, L.I.; Rabaan, A.A.; Adewumi, F.A.; Okolie, O.J.; Folorunso, J.B.; Bakhrebah, M.A.; Garout, M.; Alfouzan, W.A.; Halwani, M.A.; Alamri, A.A.; et al. Global prevalence of colistin resistance in *Klebsiella pneumoniae* from bloodstream infection: A systematic review and meta-analysis. *Pathogens* **2022**, *11*, 1092. [CrossRef]
28. March, G.A.; Bratos, M.A. A meta-analysis of in vitro antibiotic synergy against *Acinetobacter baumannii*. *J. Microbiol. Methods* **2015**, *119*, 31–36. [CrossRef]
29. Isenberg. Synergism Testing: Broth Microdilution Checkerboard and Broth Macrodilution Methods. In *Clinical Microbiology Procedures Handbook*, 4th ed.; Wiley: Hoboken, NJ, USA, 2016; Volume 1–3, pp. 5.16.1–5.16.23.
30. Lenhard, J.R.; Nation, R.L.; Tsuji, B.T. Synergistic combinations of polymyxins. *Int. J. Antimicrob. Agents* **2016**, *48*, 607–613. [CrossRef]
31. Cheng, A.; Chuang, Y.C.; Sun, H.Y.; Sheng, W.H.; Yang, C.J.; Liao, C.H.; Hsueh, P.R.; Yang, J.L.; Shen, N.J.; Wang, J.T.; et al. Excess mortality associated with colistin-tigecycline compared with colistin-carbapenem combination therapy for extensively drug-resistant *Acinetobacter baumannii* bacteremia: A multicenter prospective observational study. *Crit. Care Med.* **2015**, *43*, 1194–1204. [CrossRef]
32. Kengkla, K.; Kongpakwattana, K.; Saokaew, S.; Apisarnthanarak, A.; Chaiyakunapruk, N. Comparative efficacy and safety of treatment options for MDR and XDR *Acinetobacter baumannii* infections: A systematic review and network meta-analysis. *J. Antimicrob. Chemother.* **2018**, *73*, 22–32. [CrossRef] [PubMed]
33. Scudeller, L.; Righi, E.; Chiamenti, M.; Bragantini, D.; Menchinelli, G.; Cattaneo, P.; Giske, C.G.; Lodise, T.; Sanguinetti, M.; Piddock, L.J.V.; et al. Systematic review and meta-analysis of in vitro efficacy of antibiotic combination therapy against carbapenem-resistant Gram-negative bacilli. *Int. J. Antimicrob. Agents* **2021**, *57*, 106344. [CrossRef] [PubMed]
34. Ni, W.; Shao, X.; Di, X.; Cui, J.; Wang, R.; Liu, Y. In vitro synergy of polymyxins with other antibiotics for *Acinetobacter baumannii*: A systematic review and meta-analysis. *Int. J. Antimicrob. Agents* **2015**, *45*, 8–18. [CrossRef] [PubMed]
35. Jiang, Z.; He, X.; Li, J. Synergy effect of meropenem-based combinations against *Acinetobacter baumannii*: A systematic review and meta-analysis. *Infect. Drug Resist.* **2018**, *11*, 1083–1095. [CrossRef]
36. Zusman, O.; Avni, T.; Leibovici, L.; Adler, A.; Friberg, L.; Stergiopoulou, T.; Carmeli, Y.; Paul, M. Systematic review and meta-analysis of in vitro synergy of polymyxins and carbapenems. *Antimicrob. Agents Chemother.* **2013**, *57*, 5104–5111. [CrossRef] [PubMed]
37. Laishram, S.; Pragasam, A.K.; Bakthavatchalam, Y.D.; Veeraraghavan, B. An update on technical, interpretative and clinical relevance of antimicrobial synergy testing methodologies. *Indian J. Med. Microbiol.* **2017**, *35*, 445–468. [CrossRef]
38. Abdul-Mutakabbir, J.C.; Yim, J.; Nguyen, L.; Maassen, P.T.; Stamper, K.; Shiekh, Z.; Kebriaei, R.; Shields, R.K.; Castanheira, M.; Kaye, K.S.; et al. In vitro synergy of colistin in combination with meropenem or tigecycline against carbapenem-resistant *Acinetobacter baumannii*. *Antibiotics* **2021**, *10*, 880. [CrossRef]
39. Hong, D.J.; Kim, J.O.; Lee, H.; Yoon, E.J.; Jeong, S.H.; Yong, D.; Lee, K. In vitro antimicrobial synergy of colistin with rifampicin and carbapenems against colistin-resistant *Acinetobacter baumannii* clinical isolates. *Diagn. Microbiol. Infect. Dis.* **2016**, *86*, 184–189. [CrossRef]

40. Durante-Mangoni, E.; Signoriello, G.; Andini, R.; Mattei, A.; De Cristoforo, M.; Murino, P.; Bassetti, M.; Malacarne, P.; Petrosillo, N.; Galdieri, N.; et al. Colistin and rifampicin compared with colistin alone for the treatment of serious infections due to extensively drug-resistant *Acinetobacter baumannii*: A multicenter, randomized clinical trial. *Clin. Infect. Dis.* **2013**, *57*, 349–358. [CrossRef]
41. Aydemir, H.; Akduman, D.; Piskin, N.; Comert, F.; Horuz, E.; Terzi, A.; Kokturk, F.; Ornek, T.; Celebi, G. Colistin vs. the combination of colistin and rifampicin for the treatment of carbapenem-resistant *Acinetobacter baumannii* ventilator-associated pneumonia. *Epidemiol. Infect.* **2013**, *141*, 1214–11222. [CrossRef]
42. Park, G.C.; Choi, J.A.; Jang, S.J.; Jeong, S.H.; Kim, C.M.; Choi, I.S.; Kang, S.H.; Park, G.; Moon, D.S. In vitro interactions of antibiotic combinations of colistin, tigecycline, and doripenem against extensively drug-resistant and multidrug-resistant *Acinetobacter baumannii*. *Ann. Lab. Med.* **2016**, *36*, 124–130. [CrossRef] [PubMed]
43. Li, J.; Yang, X.; Chen, L.; Duan, X.; Jiang, Z. In vitro activity of various antibiotics in combination with tigecycline against *Acinetobacter baumannii*: A systematic review and meta-analysis. *Microb. Drug Resist.* **2017**, *23*, 982–993. [CrossRef] [PubMed]
44. Galani, I.; Orlandou, K.; Moraitou, H.; Petrikkos, G.; Souli, M. Colistin/daptomycin: An unconventional antimicrobial combination synergistic in vitro against multidrug-resistant *Acinetobacter baumannii*. *Int. J. Antimicrob. Agents* **2014**, *43*, 370–374. [CrossRef]
45. Córdoba, J.; Coronado-Álvarez, N.M.; Parra, D.; Parra-Ruiz, J. In vitro activities of novel antimicrobial combinations against extensively drug-resistant *Acinetobacter baumannii*. *Antimicrob. Agents Chemother.* **2015**, *59*, 7316–7319. [CrossRef]
46. Körber-Irrgang, B.; Kresken, M. In vitro activity of daptomycin combined with other antimicrobial agents against Gram-negative bacteria. *Clin. Microbiol. Infect.* **2010**, *16*, S156–S157.
47. Grundmann, H.; Glasner, C.; Albiger, B.; Aanensen, D.M.; Tomlinson, C.T.; Andrasević, A.T.; Cantón, R.; Carmeli, Y.; Friedrich, A.W.; Giske, C.G.; et al. Occurrence of carbapenemase-producing *Klebsiella pneumoniae* and *Escherichia coli* in the European survey of carbapenemase-producing Enterobacteriaceae (EuSCAPE): A prospective, multinational study. *Lancet Infect. Dis.* **2017**, *17*, 153–163. [CrossRef] [PubMed]
48. Maraki, S.; Mavromanolaki, V.E.; Moraitis, P.; Stafylaki, D.; Kasimati, A.; Magkafouraki, E.; Scoulica, E. Ceftazidime-avibactam, meropenen-vaborbactam, and imipenem-relebactam in combination with aztreonam against multidrug-resistant, metallo-β-lactamase-producing *Klebsiella pneumoniae*. *Eur. J. Clin. Microbiol. Infect. Dis.* **2021**, *40*, 1755–1759. [CrossRef]
49. Emeraud, C.; Escaut, L.; Boucly, A.; Fortineau, N.; Bonnin, R.A.; Naas, T.; Dortet, L. Aztreonam plus clavulanate, tazobactam, or avibactam for treatment of infections caused by metallo-β-lactamase-producing Gram-negative bacteria. *Antimicrob. Agents Chemother.* **2019**, *63*, e00010-19. [CrossRef]
50. Wenzler, E.; Deraedt, M.F.; Harrington, A.T.; Danizger, L.H. Synergistic activity of ceftazidime-avibactam and aztreonam against serine and metallo-β-lactamase-producing gram-negative pathogens. *Diagn. Microbiol. Infect. Dis.* **2017**, *88*, 352–354. [CrossRef]
51. Davido, B.; Fellous, L.; Lawrence, C.; Maxime, V.; Rottman, M.; Dinh, A. Ceftazidime-avibactam and aztreonam, an interesting strategy to overcome β-lactam resistance conferred by metallo-β-lactamases in *Enterobacteriaceae* and *Pseudomonas aeruginosa*. *Antimicrob. Agents Chemother.* **2017**, *61*, e01008-17. [CrossRef]
52. Marshall, S.; Hujer, A.M.; Rojas, L.J.; Papp-Wallace, K.M.; Humphries, R.M.; Spellberg, B.; Hujer, K.M.; Marshall, E.K.; Rudin, S.D.; Perez, F.; et al. Can ceftazidime-avibactam and aztreonam overcome β-lactam resistance conferred by metallo-β-lactamases in *Enterobacteriaceae*? *Antimicrob. Agents Chemother.* **2017**, *61*, e02243-16. [CrossRef] [PubMed]
53. Biagi, M.; Wu, T.; Lee, M.; Patel, S.; Butler, D.; Wenzler, E. Searching for the optimal treatment for metallo- and serine-β-Lactamase producing *Enterobacteriaceae*: Aztreonam in combination with ceftazidime-avibactam or meropenem-vaborbactam. *Antimicrob. Agents Chemother.* **2019**, *63*, e01426-19. [CrossRef]
54. Karakonstantis, S.; Kritsotakis, E.I.; Gikas, A. Treatment options for *K. pneumoniae*, *P. aeruginosa* and *A. baumannii* co-resistant to carbapenems, aminoglycosides, polymyxins and tigecycline: An approach based on the mechanisms of resistance to carbapenems. *Infection* **2020**, *48*, 835–851. [CrossRef]
55. Jayol, A.; Nordmann, P.; Poirel, L.; Dubois, V. Ceftazidime/avibactam alone or in combination with aztreonam against colistin-resistant and carbapenemase-producing *Klebsiella pneumoniae*. *J. Antimicrob. Chemother.* **2018**, *73*, 542–544. [CrossRef] [PubMed]
56. Falcone, M.; Daikos, G.L.; Tiseo, G.; Bassoulis, D.; Giordano, C.; Galfo, V.; Leonildi, A.; Tagliaferri, E.; Barnini, S.; Sani, S.; et al. Efficacy of ceftazidime-avibactam plus aztreonam in patients with bloodstream infections caused by metallo-β-lactamase-producing Enterobacterales. *Clin. Infect. Dis.* **2021**, *72*, 1871–1878. [CrossRef] [PubMed]
57. Mauri, C.; Maraolo, A.E.; Di Bella, S.; Luzzaro, F.; Principe, L. The revival of aztreonam in combination with avibactam against metallo-β-lactamase-producing Gram-negatives: A systematic review of in vitro studies and clinical cases. *Antibiotics* **2021**, *10*, 1012. [CrossRef] [PubMed]
58. Sader, H.S.; Carvalhaes, C.G.; Arends, S.J.R.; Castanheira, M.; Mendes, R.E. Aztreonam/avibactam activity against clinical isolates of Enterobacterales collected in Europe, Asia and Latin America in 2019. *J. Antimicrob. Chemother.* **2021**, *76*, 659–666. [CrossRef] [PubMed]
59. Rossolini, G.M.; Stone, G.; Kantecki, M.; Arhin, F.F. In vitro activity of aztreonam/avibactam against isolates of Enterobacterales collected globally from ATLAS in 2019. *J. Glob. Antimicrob. Resist.* **2022**, *30*, 214–221. [CrossRef]
60. Paul, M.; Daikos, G.L.; Durante-Mangoni, E.; Yahav, D.; Carmeli, Y.; Benattar, Y.D.; Skiada, A.; Andini, R.; Eliakim-Raz, N.; Nutman, A.; et al. Colistin alone versus colistin plus meropenem for treatment of severe infections caused by carbapenem-resistant Gram-negative bacteria: An open-label, randomised controlled trial. *Lancet Infect. Dis.* **2018**, *18*, 391–400. [CrossRef]

61. Gutiérrez-Gutiérrez, B.; Salamanca, E.; de Cueto, M.; Hsueh, P.R.; Viale, P.; Paño-Pardo, J.R.; Venditti, M.; Tumbarello, M.; Daikos, G.; Cantón, R.; et al. Effect of appropriate combination therapy on mortality of patients with bloodstream infections due to carbapenemase-producing Enterobacteriaceae (INCREMENT): A retrospective cohort study. *Lancet Infect. Dis.* **2017**, *17*, 726–734. [CrossRef]
62. Liu, Q.; Li, W.; Feng, Y.; Tao, C. Efficacy and safety of polymyxins for the treatment of *Acinectobacter baumannii* infection: A systematic review and meta-analysis. *PLoS ONE* **2014**, *9*, e98091. [CrossRef] [PubMed]
63. Dickstein, Y.; Lellouche, J.; Ben Dalak Amar, M.; Schwartz, D.; Nutman, A.; Daitch, V.; Yahav, D.; Leibovici, L.; Skiada, A.; Antoniadou, A.; et al. Treatment outcomes of colistin- and carbapenem-resistant *Acinetobacter baumannii* infections: An exploratory subgroup analysis of a randomized clinical trial. *Clin. Infect. Dis.* **2019**, *69*, 769–776. [CrossRef] [PubMed]
64. Karakonstantis, S.; Ioannou, P.; Samonis, G.; Kofteridis, D.P. Systematic review of antimicrobial combination options for pandrug-resistant *Acinetobacter baumannii*. *Antibiotics* **2021**, *10*, 1344. [CrossRef] [PubMed]
65. Perez, F.; El Chakhtoura, N.G.; Yasmin, M.; Bonomo, R.A. Polymyxins: To combine or not to combine? *Antibiotics* **2019**, *8*, 38. [CrossRef] [PubMed]
66. Pillai, S.K.; Moellering, R.C.; Eliopoulos, G.M. Antimicrobial combinations. In *Antimicrobials in Laboratory Medicine*, 5th ed.; Lippincott Williams & Wilkins: Philadelphia, PA, USA, 2005; pp. 365–435.

antibiotics

MDPI

Article

Curcumin Stimulates the Overexpression of Virulence Factors in *Salmonella enterica* Serovar Typhimurium: In Vitro and Animal Model Studies

Martin Zermeño-Ruiz [1], Itzia A. Rangel-Castañeda [2], Daniel Osmar Suárez-Rico [3], Leonardo Hernández-Hernández [3], Rafael Cortés-Zárate [1], José M. Hernández-Hernández [2], Gabriela Camargo-Hernández [4] and Araceli Castillo-Romero [1,*]

[1] Departamento de Microbiología y Patología, Centro Universitario de Ciencias de la Salud, Universidad de Guadalajara, Calle Sierra Mojada 950, Independencia Oriente, Guadalajara 44100, Mexico
[2] Centro de Investigación y Estudios Avanzados del Instituto Politécnico Nacional, Ciudad de México 07360, Mexico
[3] Departamento de Fisiología, Centro Universitario de Ciencias de la Salud, Universidad de Guadalajara, Calle Sierra Mojada 950, Independencia Oriente, Guadalajara 44100, Mexico
[4] Departamento de Ciencias de la Salud, Centro Universitario de los Altos, Universidad de Guadalajara, Av. Rafael Casillas Aceves No. 1200, Tepatitlán de Morelos 44100, Mexico
* Correspondence: araceli.castillo@academicos.udg.mx

Abstract: *Salmonella* spp. is one of the most common food poisoning pathogens and the main cause of diarrheal diseases in humans in developing countries. The increased *Salmonella* resistance to antimicrobials has led to the search for new alternatives, including natural compounds such as curcumin, which has already demonstrated a bactericidal effect; however, in Gram-negatives, there is much controversy about this effect, as it is highly variable. In this study, we aimed to verify the antibacterial activity of curcumin against the *Salmonella enterica* serovar Typhimurium growth rate, virulence, and pathogenicity. The strain was exposed to 110, 220 or 330 μg/mL curcumin, and by complementary methods (spectrophotometric, pour plate and MTT assays), we determined its antibacterial activity. To elucidate whether curcumin regulates the expression of virulence genes, *Salmonella invA*, *fliC* and *siiE* genes were investigated by quantitative real-time reverse transcription (qRT-PCR). Furthermore, to explore the effect of curcumin on the pathogenesis process in vivo, a *Caenorhabditis elegans* infection model was employed. No antibacterial activity was observed, even at higher concentrations of curcumin. All concentrations of curcumin caused overgrowth (35–69%) and increased the pathogenicity of the bacterial strain through the overexpression of virulence factors. The latter coincided with a significant reduction in both the lifespan and survival time of *C. elegans* when fed with curcumin-treated bacteria. Our data provide relevant information that may support the selective antibacterial effects of curcumin to reconsider the indiscriminate use of this phytochemical, especially in outbreaks of pathogenic Gram-negative bacteria.

Keywords: *Salmonella enterica* serovar Typhimurium; curcumin; antibacterial activity; pathogenicity; *C. elegans*

1. Introduction

Diarrheal disease is an important global health problem and is the third cause of child mortality [1]. *Salmonella* is one of the most frequent bacteria causing diarrheal diseases [2]. *Salmonella enterica* serotypes include numerous pathogens of warm-blooded animals, including humans. *Salmonella enterica* serovar Typhimurium (*S.* Typhimurium) has been considered the prototypical broad-host-range serotype. It is a frequent cause of acute self-limiting food-borne diarrhea in numerous species, including humans, livestock, domestic fowl, rodents, and birds [3]. Recently, nontyphoidal *Salmonella* variants were associated with invasive systemic disease and high mortality rates within immunocompromised patients. *S.* Typhimurium and Enteritidis are the most usual causes of invasive disease in sub-Saharan Africa [4,5]. The pathogenicity of *Salmonella enterica* infections is expressed in three ways, such as host cell invasion, intracellular survival, and colonization. All these processes are regulated by the virulence genes located in *Salmonella* pathogenicity islands (SPI). The most extensive invasion mechanism requires the type III secretion system encoded in the SPI-1. This system is composed of a needle-like structure that injects bacterial effector proteins into epithelial cells, such as the invasion protein A (InvA). InvA is widely studied as a virulence factor; it is required to cross the epithelial cells, thus initiating infection [6,7]. Another entry mechanism involved bacterial motility. Recent data demonstrated that the deletion of flagellin gene *fliC*, which encodes the major component of the flagellum in *S.* Typhimurium, affects the entry of *Salmonella* into the host cell [8,9]. In addition, novel members of the non-fimbrial adhesins encoded in SPI-4 have been found. In a murine model, SPI-4 contributed to intestinal inflammation, via the secretion of SiiE that mediates the *Salmonella* adhesion to the epithelial cell's surface [10].

Specific antimicrobial therapy ameliorates the course of illness with these pathogens. However, because of the problem of antibiotic resistance, alternative approaches have been directed toward therapies based on traditional plant medicines.

Due to its multi-faceted pharmacology, many studies have evaluated the possible use of curcumin (CUR) to treat or prevent bacterial infections. Several studies showed this phytochemical, alone or combined with some nanomaterials or compounds, demonstrated different responses of curcumin on Gram-positive and Gram-negative bacteria. In Gram-negative bacteria, curcumin exhibits extremely low antibacterial activity [11–22]. In addition, Marathe and coworkers (2010) proved in a murine model that CUR enhances the pathogenicity of *S.* Typhimurium via regulating their defense pathways [23]. While there appear to be countless therapeutic benefits to curcumin, its effects on Gram-negative bacteria are still poorly understood and controversial.

On the other hand, the *Caenorhabditis elegans* genome can encode several antimicrobial proteins, such as caenopores, lysozymes, lectins and ABF peptides (antibacterial factors), that have a broad antimicrobial spectrum for Gram-positive bacteria [24]. Additionally, the finding that diverse bacteria are pathogenic to *C. elegans* opens the prospect of using this experimentally simple model to study microbial pathogenesis [25]. In this work, we described the role of CUR in the pathogenicity of *S.* Typhimurium. Our results demonstrated that CUR increases cell proliferation and induces *S.* Typhimurium virulence factors overexpression. Consequently, the lifespan of *C. elegans* was reduced.

2. Results

2.1. PCR Identification of Genes Encoding Specific Virulence Factors of S. Typhimurium

Virulence factors are essential for the ability of bacteria to cause disease. *Salmonella* has the ability to survive long-term frozen storage; however, it has been reported that isolated virulent bacterial strains became avirulent during storage or passages. The above is probably due to the loss of virulence plasmids [26]. A polymerase chain reaction (PCR) method confirmed that our storage and growth conditions did not affect the presence of virulence factors from the bacterial strain. Figure 1 shows the presence of three genes of *S.* Typhimurium involved in epithelial cell adhesion and invasion (*invA*, *fliC* and *siiE*).

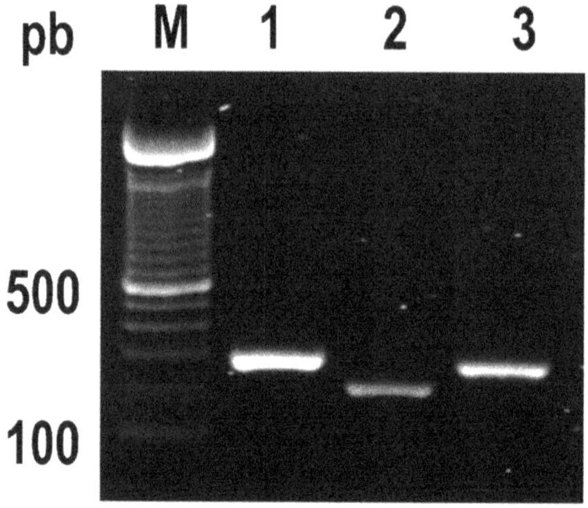

Figure 1. PCR detection of *Salmonella* Typhimurium virulence genes. Lane 1, *invA* gene (1322 bp). Lane 2, *siiE* gene (240 bp), and Lane 3 *fliC* gene (307 bp). M, DNA ladder, standard molecular size marker.

2.2. Curcumin Did Not Show an Antibacterial Effect

To determine whether CUR kills *S.* Typhimurium and to investigate the effect of different environmental or growth conditions on bacteria cell survival, 10^7 CFU/mL was exposed to dimethyl sulfoxide (DMSO) or CUR for 2 h, and the effect was evaluated by spectrophotometric (OD600), pour plate and MTT assay. The results, presented in Figure 2, indicate that the treatment with 110, 220 and 330 µg/mL of CUR did not inhibit bacterial growth. After 4 h of incubation, curcumin provoked a significant dose-dependent growth stimulation. Untreated and DMSO-treated Salmonella strains reached the exponential growth phase with similar growth rate (Figure 2A). After 12 h of incubation, *Salmonella* maintained a significant growth increase in the presence of CUR (DMSO 3.6 ± 0.09 SD vs 110 µg/mL 3.8 ± 0.05 SD, 220 µg/mL 4.6 ± 0.06 SD and 330 µg/mL 4.9 ± 0.04 SD) (Figure 2B). By the pour plate, there was an increment in the number of colonies with CUR following a dose-response profile (Table 1, Figure 3A). The percentage of overgrowth in *S.* Typhimurium increased significantly from 35% to 57% (Figure 3B). These results are consistent with the MTT assay, where formazan cell viability/crystal formation increases with curcumin concentrations. When formazan was solubilized, the absorbance at 550 nm of curcumin-treated cultures was higher than the negative controls, maintaining the dose-dependent profile (DSMO 0.1925 ± 0.004 vs 110 µg/mL 0.2095 ± 0.01, 220 µg/mL 0.2297 ± 0.04, 330 µg/mL 0.2758 ± 0.018) (Figure 4).

Table 1. Number of colonies on agar plates.

Sample	[A] Average Number of Colonies Per Milliliter with Dilution 10^4
	S. Typhimurium
Untreated	1.30×10^7 CFU/mL
DMSO	1.13×10^7 CFU/mL
CUR 110 µg/mL	1.52×10^7 CFU/mL
CUR 220 µg/mL	1.72×10^7 CFU/mL
CUR 330 µg/mL	1.77×10^7 CFU/mL

[A] six replicates.

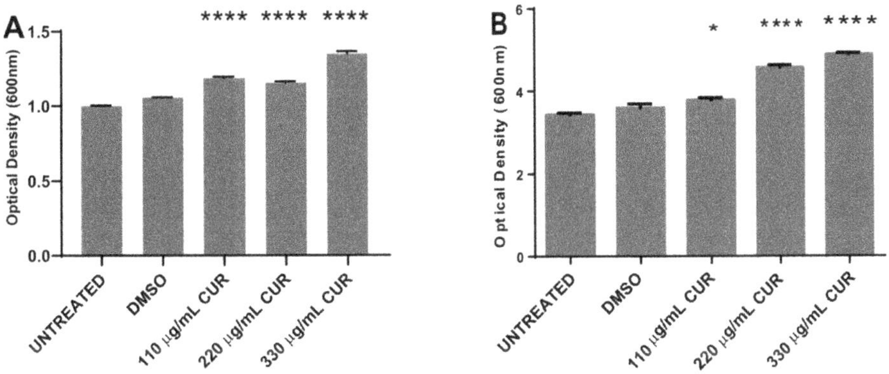

Figure 2. Dose–time response curves comparing curcumin (CUR) treatment in *S. enterica* ser. Typhimurium growth (OD600), and for cells incubated in the presence of dimethyl sulfoxide (DMSO). Curves are representative of at least 3 different assays. (**A**) After 4 h of incubation. (**B**) After 12 h of incubation. (* $p < 0.05$, **** $p < 0.0001$).

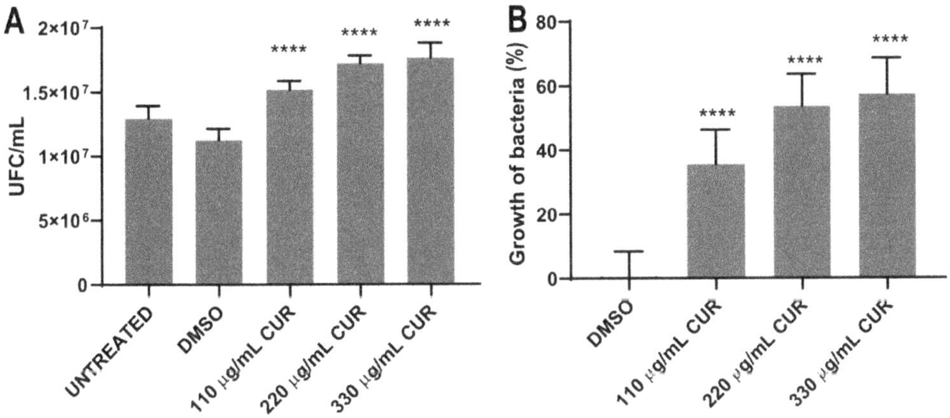

Figure 3. Number of colonies on agar plates (**A**) and percentage growth of *S. enterica* ser. Typhimurium (**B**), after treatment with CUR. The average and standard deviation values of six replicates are shown for the strain. (**** $p < 0.0001$).

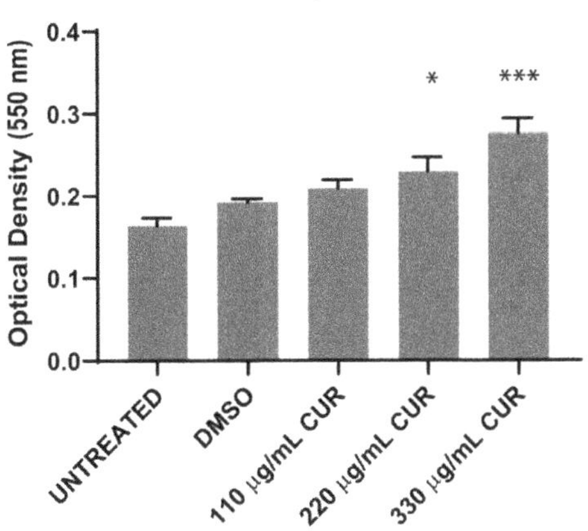

Figure 4. MTT reduction by *S. enterica* ser. Typhimurium treated with CUR, (* $p < 0.05$, *** $p < 0.001$).

2.3. Virulence Factors Are Upregulated by Curcumin

It has been demonstrated that CUR attenuates the virulence pathogens by the down-regulation of transcription of virulence genes [27,28]. We measured *fliC*, *siiE* and *invA* expression levels by relative–quantitative RT-PCR to determine whether CUR directly affected bacterial virulence. All genes showed significant gene expression changes in response to CUR treatment. In *S.* Typhimurium, treatment with CUR provoked the increase in mRNA expression for *siiE*, *invA* and *fliC*. Among the three genes, *siiE* had the higher range of mRNA expression (18- and 28-fold), with the concentrations of 220 and 330 μg/mL of CUR, respectively (Figure 5A), while *invA* had the smallest range (0.4- and 0.9-fold), with the same doses (Figure 5B). Finally, *fliC* had also significantly increased mRNA expression (5- and 10-fold) with 220 and 330 μg/mL of CUR, respectively (Figure 5C).

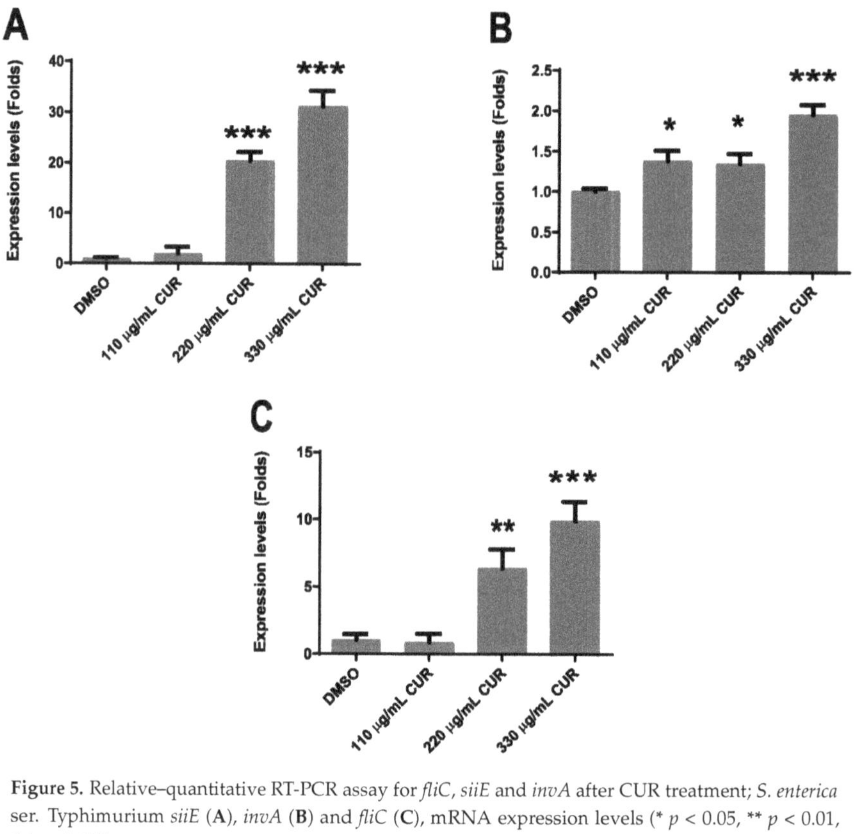

Figure 5. Relative–quantitative RT-PCR assay for *fliC*, *siiE* and *invA* after CUR treatment; *S. enterica* ser. Typhimurium *siiE* (**A**), *invA* (**B**) and *fliC* (**C**), mRNA expression levels (* $p < 0.05$, ** $p < 0.01$, *** $p < 0.001$).

2.4. Curcumin Enhanced the Pathogenicity of S. Typhimurium in C. elegans

Earlier reports have shown that *S.* Typhimurium can kill *C. elegans* [24,29]. To validate nematode survival in the presence of this pathogenic strain, 8×10^8 cells/mL were used as bacterial food for *C. elegans*, and nematode survival was evaluated. As a negative control, nematodes fed with *E. coli* OP50 were used. The results obtained show that the mean and maximum life expectancy of nematodes fed with the pathogenic strain decreased significantly, with respect to worms fed with the OP50 strain (negative control) (Figure 6A). To validate whether CUR increased the virulence of *Salmonella*, 8×10^8 cells/mL were exposed for 2 h to DMSO and 110 and 330 μg/mL of CUR, and subsequently used as nematode food. The results show that feeding *C. elegans* with CUR-treated bacteria significantly shortens the lifespan of the nematode by 66% at the 330 μg/mL concentration compared to DMSO treatment (Figure 6B). The above effect correlates with the overexpression of virulence factors in *S.* Typhimurium due to the use of CUR. Survival curve of worms fed with DMSO-treated bacteria were not different from the curve of worms fed with untreated bacteria (Figure 6, LogRank $p = 0.968$ for *S.* Typhimurium, n = 90). OP50-fed worms showed the usual lifespan, ranging from 16 to 22 days.

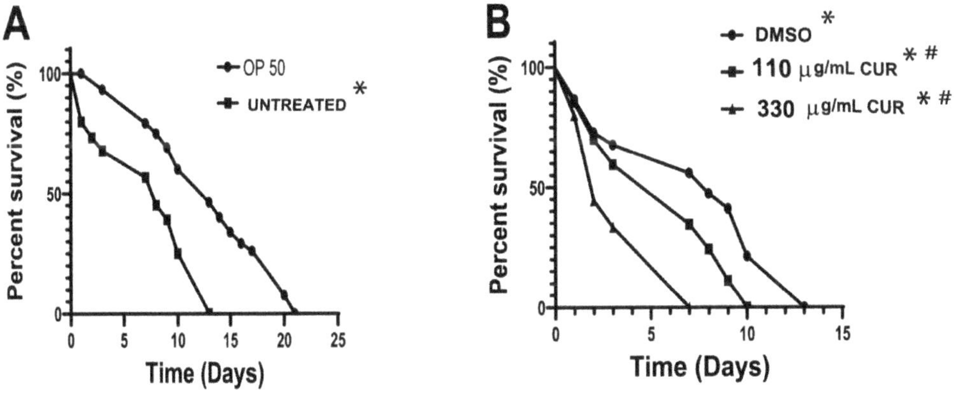

Figure 6. Lifespan of C. elegans infected with *S. enterica* ser. Typhimurium strain treated with 110 and 330 μg/mL of CUR (**A**). Survival curves for nematodes fed with *S.* Typhimurium and *Escherichia coli* OP50. (**B**) Life expectancy of nematodes fed with *S.* Typhimurium pretreated with DMSO, 110 and 330 μg/mL. Kaplan–Meier survival curves for *S. enterica* ser. Typhimurium. Survival percent are based on data from pathogenicity assay. Data were analyzed by log rank test, and all pairwise multiple comparison procedures used the Holm–Sidak method. n = 90, * $p < 0.001$ in relation to the OP50 and # $p < 0.001$ regarding the Untreated.

3. Discussion

Diarrheal diseases are one of the leading causes of death in children under 5 years and adults over 65 years. After Rotavirus, enteric bacteria are an important cause of morbidity and mortality. *S.* Typhimurium is included among the major isolated agents in developing countries [1,30]. Antibiotics are effective in life-threatening cases caused by bacterial pathogens; however, due to increased resistance and the potentially serious side effects of combinatorial therapies, there is a pressing need to have new alternatives [31–34]. In recent years, CUR, the principal and most active curcuminoid of *Curcuma longa* L. (*C. longa*), has gained considerable attention, due to its antimicrobial activity in different strains of bacteria. In 2016, Hayati Gunes et al [19] found that CUR has high antibacterial activity against *E. coli*, in relation to other bacteria, with a minimum inhibitory concentration (MIC) for CUR of 163 μg/mL. Others found that in combination with antibiotics, the CUR antibacterial activity ranges from 125 to 500 μg/mL [35]. Although most studies suggest that CUR has activity against both Gram-positive and Gram-negative bacteria [11–13,16–21], its activity against *S.* Typhimurium is considerably controversial. Meanwhile, in chicken, treatment with *C. longa* prevents intestinal colonization by *S.* Typhimurium [36]. In a murine model, CUR increases the pathogenicity of this bacteria [23]. In addition, reports are showing that the efficacy of antibiotics is directly related to the level of inoculum size. Bacteria might appear susceptible when the inoculum is low density (10^5 CFU/mL) but resistant if the inoculum size is increased (high density ~10^9 CFU/mL; depending on the clinical strains) [37–39]. In this report, we explore the antibacterial efficacy of CUR, and the killing assay was performed using 10^7 CFU/mL. In the present study, even though we followed the procedure reported by Hayati Gunes et al. [19], CUR at 110, 220 and 330 μg/mL for 16–18 h at 37 °C, 250 rpm, was not active against *S.* Typhimurium (data not shown). It is well documented that the bacterial growth rate determines the bacterial susceptibility to antimicrobials; bacterial overgrowth provokes the nutrients deprivation that induces modifications of the cell envelope [40], and generally, there is no correlation with the antimicrobial concentration. Considering this, CUR treatment was performed throughout each phase of growth. Our results provide evidence that CUR did not inhibit the growth of *Salmonella*, but promoted a significant overgrowth instead, after 4 h of incubation. Many bacterial species and antibiotic classes exhibit heteroresistance, meaning that a susceptible bacterial isolate harbors a resistant subpopulation that can grow in the presence of an antibiotic. In this work, CUR was in contact with *Salmonella* for only 2 h, after which it was removed, but, interestingly, in *Salmonella*, the overgrowth continued after 12 h of incubation. This suggests that CUR enhances the speed at which cells proliferate and that the modification is transmitted to new generations. It has been reported that *S.* Typhimurium has some genes with diverged expression domains that are involved in different metabolic pathways compared with *E. coli*, leading to their better survival and propagation [41–43]. More studies are necessary to identify how CUR regulates the growth in *Salmonella*. On the other hand, the standard optical method for quantifying cell density (OD 600 nm) cannot distinguish live from dead bacteria or even particles. Therefore, in order to improve the results, viability and metabolic activity was validated by the pour plate method and MTT assay [44–46]. Our results confirm that, after 12 h of incubation, CUR does not affect the growth of *S.* Typhimurium; we have metabolic active growing cells.

CUR has been found to modulate the activity of several key transcription factors and, in turn, the cellular expression profiles [47]. In bacteria and parasites, CUR is reported to modulate the virulence factor expression [27,28]. The pathogenicity of bacteria is related to many and strain-specific virulence factors. In *Salmonella*, we analyzed three virulence genes, *invA* for the *Salmonella* genus, *fliC*, and *siiE* for Typhimurium serovar. Our result showed that all genes were found to be upregulated by CUR. For *invA*, a gene that mediates invasiveness, the overexpression was only 0.9-fold. The higher overexpression levels were observed with *fliC* and *siiE* (10- and 28-fold, respectively). In another *Salmonella* species, flagella could be dispensable for host cell adhesion, but for *S.* Typhimurium, the flagellum is a key virulence-associated phenotype. A functional flagellum is necessary for epithelial cell invasion and macrophage uptake; besides, it participates in proinflammatory cytokine expression. In the case of the adhesin SIIE, some studies show that the infection of host organisms by *Salmonella* involves the cooperative activity of the *Salmonella* pathogenicity island 1 (SPI1)-encoded type III secretion system (T3SS) and SIIE. Without the function of the SPI4 T1SS or SiiE, *Salmonella* is highly reduced in adhesion [7,48,49]. Our results suggest that CUR enhances the adhesion ability of *Salmonella*. Further studies are needed to elucidate the exact mechanism by which CUR upregulates the expression of the major virulence factors of *S.* Typhimurium [23,50,51]. The higher pathogenic potential, which bacterial strains exposed to CUR possess, was validated using the nematode *C. elegans*. It is known that *S.* Typhimurium is pathogenic to *C. elegans*; even though the nematode expresses numerous antimicrobial proteins, this bacterial strain proliferates and establishes a persistent infection in the intestine of the nematode [52]. In this study, the overexpression of virulence factors in *Salmonella* by CUR correlates with the short lifespans of *C. elegans* in a lifespan assay. The rate of mortality of *C. elegans* fed with untreated *S.* Typhimurium was similar to that found by other authors [25]; the life expectancy of the nematode was reduced by 66%, in comparison to the *E. coli* OP50 strain. In nematodes fed with CUR-treated *S.* Typhimurium, there was a direct correlation between the overexpression of virulence genes and the mortality rate; the complete mortality occurred after 10 and 7 days with 110 and 330 μg/mL, respectively, suggesting increased bacterial infection after exposure to CUR. In contrast, with other Gram-negative bacteria, it has been reported that CUR reduced the production of virulence factors, affecting the adherence and the formation of biofilm [28]. It is important to emphasize that further studies are necessary.

4. Materials and Methods

4.1. Bacterial Strain

Dr. Jeannette Barba León, Universidad de Guadalajara, kindly provided the *S.* Typhimurium (071M7) used in the current study [53].

4.2. Maintenance and Preservation of Microorganisms

The bacterial strain was grown in nutritive agar (plates) (Becton Dickinson, Maryland, USA) at 37 °C for 18–20 h. The cultures were stored at 4 °C, with streak plating onto fresh agar plates every seven days. A glycerol stock of bacteria was stored at −80 °C.

4.3. Extraction of Genomic DNA

Genomic DNA was obtained from *S.* Typhimurium cultures using the DNeasy® Blood & Tissue kit (QIAGEN, Hilden, Germany), following the manufacturer's instructions. The DNA was stored at −20 °C. Purity and concentration were determined by 1% agarose (Ultra-Pure—Agarose, Invitrogen, Carlsbad, CA, USA) gel electrophoresis and by spectrophotometry, respectively. Electrophoretic gels were stained with GelRed (Nucleic Acid Gel, Biotium, Landing Pkwy, CA, USA) and visualized on a trans-illuminator (UVP Benchtop 2UV, Fisher Scientific, Waltham, MA, USA).

4.4. Presence of Virulence Genes

The pathogenicity of *Salmonella* spp. has been related to numerous virulence genes. The invasion protein InvA is one of the most studied virulence factors. Flic-encoded flagellin protein, and the giant, non-fimbrial adhesin protein SIIE have been also implicated in successful host infection [10,54,55]. The expression of *invA* (GenBank Accession M90846.1), *fliC* (GenBank Accession KF589316.1) and *siiE* (GenBank Accession AJ576316.1) was validated in the bacterial strain. A specific region of each gene was amplified from genomic DNA (DNeasy® Blood & Tissue, IAGEN) by PCR using the following primers: *siiE* sense 5′-CGA CCT GAG TCA CCG TTG GGC GAT-3 and *siiE* antisense 5′- ATT GGG CTC GGC ACT GCC ACT 3′(210 bp), *invA* sense 5′- ATG CCG GTG AAA TTA TCG CCA CGT-3′, *invA* antisense 5′- ATG CCG GCA ATA GCG TCA CCT-3′(322 bp), fliC sense 5′-AAA GCC TCG GCT ACT GGT CTT GGT G -3′ and *fliC* antisense 5′- ATG CTG TGC CGG TAA CAC CTG CTG-3′(307 bp). The PCR conditions were 95 °C for 60 s, 37 cycles at 95 °C for 30 s, 72 °C for 60 s and 72 °C for 7 min. The resulting amplicons were visualized by electrophoresis in 1% agarose gel.

4.5. Preparation of Curcumin Stocks

The CUR was acquired from Sigma-Aldrich (≥65% (HPLC), St Louis, MO, USA). CUR stock was prepared using dimethyl sulfoxide (1.2% DMSO, Sigma-Aldrich) as a diluent and then diluted to a final concentration of 110, 220 and 330 µg/mL in phosphate-buffered saline (PBS) [56].

4.6. Determination of the Antibacterial Activity of Curcumin

4.6.1. Spectrophotometric Method

The antibacterial activity of CUR was determined by a growing strain in Luria Bertani broth (LB) (Sigma-Aldrich, Missouri, USA), at 37 °C, 250 rpm. Cultures were allowed to grow until they reached OD600 0.08 (10^7 colony forming units CFU/mL). Cells were pelleted by centrifugation at 1844× g for 5 min (Sigma 1-14K 12092 rotor), resuspended in 3 mL of PBS containing 110, 220 and 330 µg/mL of CUR and incubated for 2 h at 37 °C, 250 rpm. Untreated and 1.2% DMSO-treated cultures were used as negative controls. After the incubation period, cells were harvested by centrifugation, washed with PBS twice to remove the CUR, and grown in LB medium to achieve the exponential phase [18]. Bacterial growth (OD600) in LB medium was measured on a microplate reader (BioTek Synergy HT, Winooski, VT, USA). All experiments were performed in triplicate.

4.6.2. Pour Plate Method

S. Typhimurium strain was exposed to DMSO, 110, 220 or 330 µg/mL of CUR for 2 h following the procedure described above. After CUR treatment, cells were harvested by centrifugation as mentioned above. The pellets were resuspended in 3 mL of PBS, and serial dilutions were performed. For the pour plate method, 100 µL of each dilution was added by pipette to the center of sterile disposable Petri dishes. Then, cooled but still molten agar medium was poured into each Petri dish. The plates were incubated overnight at 37 °C. The dilutions chosen produced between 30 and 300 separate countable colonies. The growth percentage was calculated as ((B2-A2)/A2 100)), where A is the number of colonies untreated, and B is the number of colonies in the presence of CUR. All experiments were performed in triplicate.

4.6.3. Assay MTT

According to previous reports, MTT assay modified by Wang et al. [44] was performed to determine the viability of *S.* Typhimurium after DMSO, 0, 110, 220 or 330 µg/mL of CUR exposition. Briefly, a bacterial strain was grown at 37 °C in LB broth until the OD600 reached 0.1, and then DMSO or CUR was added to each cell culture. After incubation for 2 h at 37 °C at 250 rpm, cultures were centrifuged at 1844× *g* for 5 min (Sigma 1-14K 12092 rotor). The resulting bacterial pellets were washed three times in PBS and resuspended in 1 mL of LB. Aliquots of the bacterial cultures (20 µL) were placed on 0.6 mL tubes, which had been preheated to 37 °C for 10 min. Then, 2 µL of MTT (5 mg/mL, Sigma-Aldrich, M5655 St Louis, MO, USA) was added to each tube. After incubation, for 20 min at 37 °C, the tubes were centrifuged at 10,000× *g* for 1 min (Sigma 1-14K 12092 rotor) in order to precipitate the bacteria and formazan crystals; 20 µL of the medium was removed, and the crystals were dissolved with 250 µL of DMSO. Finally, the coloration was read at 550 nm after 15 min in a microplate reader (BioTek Synergy HT, Winooski, VT, USA). All experiments were performed in triplicate.

4.6.4. Statistical Analysis

All data were presented as mean values with standard deviations and analyzed using two-way ANOVA, followed by Dunnett's multiple comparisons test (GraphPad Prism version 6.01 for Windows, GraphPad Software, La Jolla, CA, USA). p-values of $\leq$0.05 were considered significantly different.

4.7. Relative-Quantitative RT-PCR

The effect of CUR on the expression of *invA*, *fliC* and *siiE*, genes associated with the virulence of *S.* Typhimurium, was evaluated by semi-quantitative qRT-PCR using the primers described above. First, the bacteria strain was exposed to DMSO, 110, 220 or 330 µg/mL of CUR for 2 h following the procedure described above. After CUR remotion, they were grown overnight in LB medium. Total RNA was obtained from DMSO, or CUR treated bacterial cultures using a Total RNA Purification kit (NORGEN), following the manufacturer's instructions. cDNAs were synthesized by a reverse transcriptase reaction (Verso cDNA Synthesis Kit, Thermo Scientific) using 1 µg of RNA and Oligo dt20 primer (Integrated DNA). Relative–quantitative RT-PCR was performed in a StepOneTM Real-Time PCR System (Applied Biosystems™, Foster City, CA, USA) using Maxima SYBR Green qPCR Master Mix (Thermo Scientific) to evaluate the amplification reaction. The gene expression was normalized to the expression level of glyceraldehyde 3-phosphate dehydrogenase genes (GenBank accession no. DQ644683.1) using the following primers: gapdh sense 5′- GGT TTT GGC CGT ATC GGT CGC A-3′ and gapdh antisense 5′- ACC GGT AGC TTC AGC CAC TAC G-3′. Melting curves confirmed the absence of primer dimerization. The amplification conditions were as follows: hot start at 95 °C 10 min, 40 cycles of 95 °C 15 s, 60 °C 30 s and 72 °C 30 s. The comparative ΔΔCt method calculated changes in expression [57]. Significant differences (defined as $p < 0.05$, indicated by asterisks in figures) were calculated by ANOVA tests using the GraphPad Prism version 6.01 for

Windows (GraphPad Software, La Jolla, CA, USA). Error bars indicate standard deviations for experiments with more than one trial.

4.8. Maintenance and Preservation of C. elegans

The wild-type *C. elegans* variety Bristol N2 strain used in this study was provided by the Caenorhabditis Genetics Center (CGC, Minneapolis, MN, USA). Adult worms were used for all experiments, age-synchronized according to standard methods. Nematodes were grown and maintained monoxenically at 20 °C, on nematode growth medium (NGM) [58]. Animals were grown on Petri plates seeded with *Escherichia coli* strain OP50 as a food source [59,60].

4.9. Pathogenicity Assays of Salmonella Strains on the C. elegans Model

A pathogenicity assay is a lifespan assay, where *C. elegans* strains on NGM agar plates are fed with pathogenic bacteria (known here as killing plates) instead of the regular *E. coli* OP50 [29]. In this study, *S.* Typhimurium was grown overnight in LB at 37 °C, 250 rpm and then resuspended at an OD600 = 1. Then, cells were harvested by centrifugation, and the pellets were resuspended in 3 mL of PBS containing DMSO, 110 or 330 μg/mL of CUR and incubated for 2 h at 37 °C, 250 rpm. The killing plates were prepared by dropping 10 μL of bacterial suspension (8×10^8 CFU/mL) onto NGM agar plates and incubated for 16 h at room temperature [61]. After that, 30 age-synchronized L4 worms were transferred to the killing plates. Since *C. elegans* starts laying eggs on day 1 of adulthood, the worms were transferred to fresh killing plates from the 2nd to 14th days to prevent a mistaken offspring score. In the remaining days of the trial, the transfers were carried out within a longer time (when food ran out) because the worms were in the non-reproductive phase. Worms that were alive, dead, or missing were determined and counted every other day along the time course of dying for the population, using a touch movement assay for death [62]. This assay consists of visually inspecting the worm for movement; if there is movement, then it scored as alive, and if there is no movement, even when its body is gently touched with a worm picker, it is scored as dead. Missing worms, those lost or burrowing into the medium or climbing the plate walls and drying up, were censored from the analysis. NGM agar plates seeded with untreated *S.* Typhimurium and *E. coli* OP50 were used as positive and negative controls. Every experiment was repeated three times. Data were analyzed using the Kaplan–Meier survival test and weighted log-rank tests [63]. Actual P-values are included in the figures; asterisks indicate significant differences. Differences were considered significant at $p < 0.05$.

5. Conclusions

This research provides new evidence on the antibacterial activity of CUR against one of the major enteric bacterial pathogens, *Salmonella*. We demonstrated that CUR increases the cell proliferation of *S.* Typhimurium, and we also observed a deregulation of three genes involved in the pathogenicity of *S.* Typhimurium leading to an increase in virulence in agreement with the results of in vivo assays. These results urge us to reconsider the indiscriminate use of CUR, especially in outbreaks of pathogenic Gram-negative bacteria.

Author Contributions: Conceptualization, L.H.-H., R.C.-Z. and A.C.-R.; Formal analysis, M.Z.-R. and L.H.-H.; Funding acquisition, I.A.R.-C., L.H.-H., R.C.-Z. and A.C.-R.; Investigation, M.Z.-R. and A.C.-R.; Methodology, M.Z.-R., I.A.R.-C., D.O.S.-R., L.H.-H., J.M.H.-H., G.C.-H. and A.C.-R.; Project administration, A.C.-R.; Supervision, A.C.-R.; Writing—original draft, M.Z.-R.; Writing—review and editing, I.A.R.-C., D.O.S.-R., L.H.-H., R.C.-Z., J.M.H.-H., G.C.-H. and A.C.-R. All authors have read and agreed to the published version of the manuscript.

Funding: This research was funded by PRODEP IDCA-28301) from Secretaría de Educación Pública SEP, and partially supported by a grant (number FODECIJAL IDCA-8129) from Consejo Estatal de Ciencia y Tecnología de Jalisco COECYTJAL and PIN 2021-II-CUCS from Universidad de Guadalajara.

Data Availability Statement: Not applicable.

Acknowledgments: We are grateful to the C. elegans Genetics Center (CGC), which is supported by NIH's National Center for Research Resources, for providing wild-type N2 strain. Martin Zermeño-Ruiz wants to thank Consejo Nacional de Ciencia y Tecnología (CONACYT) for fellowship no. 751855. The authors would like to thank Enago (www.enago.com) for the English language review.

Conflicts of Interest: The authors declare no conflict of interest.

References

1. Troeger, C.; Blacker, B.F.; Khalil, I.A.; Rao, P.C.; Cao, S.; Zimsen, S.R.M.; Albertson, S.B.; Stanaway, J.D.; Deshpande, A.; Abebe, Z.; et al. Estimates of the global, regional, and national morbidity, mortality, and aetiologies of diarrhoea in 195 countries: A systematic analysis for the Global Burden of Disease Study 2016. *Lancet Infect. Dis.* **2018**, *18*, 1211–1228. [CrossRef]
2. Ferrari, R.G.; Rosario, D.K.A.; Cunha-Neto, A.; Mano, S.B.; Figueiredo, E.E.S.; Conte-Junior, C.A. Worldwide Epidemiology of Salmonella Serovars in Animal-Based Foods: A Meta-analysis. *Appl. Environ. Microbiol.* **2019**, *85*, e00591-19. [CrossRef] [PubMed]
3. Rabsch, W.; Andrews, H.L.; Kingsley, R.A.; Prager, R.; Tschape, H.; Adams, L.G.; Baumler, A.J. Salmonella enterica serotype Typhimurium and its host-adapted variants. *Infect. Immun.* **2002**, *70*, 2249–2255. [CrossRef] [PubMed]
4. Kingsley, R.A.; Msefula, C.L.; Thomson, N.R.; Kariuki, S.; Holt, K.E.; Gordon, M.A.; Harris, D.; Clarke, L.; Whitehead, S.; Sangal, V.; et al. Epidemic multiple drug resistant Salmonella Typhimurium causing invasive disease in sub-Saharan Africa have a distinct genotype. *Genome Res.* **2009**, *19*, 2279–2287. [CrossRef]
5. Feasey, N.A.; Dougan, G.; Kingsley, R.A.; Heyderman, R.S.; Gordon, M.A. Invasive non-typhoidal salmonella disease: An emerging and neglected tropical disease in Africa. *Lancet* **2012**, *379*, 2489–2499. [CrossRef]
6. Imke Hansen-Wester, M.H. Salmonella pathogenicity islands encoding type III secretion systems. *Microbes Infect.* **2001**, *3*, 549–559. [CrossRef]
7. Dos Santos, A.M.P.; Ferrari, R.G.; Conte-Junior, C.A. Virulence Factors in Salmonella Typhimurium: The Sagacity of a Bacterium. *Curr. Microbiol.* **2019**, *76*, 762–773. [CrossRef]
8. Elhadad, D.; Desai, P.; Rahav, G.; McClelland, M.; Gal-Mor, O. Flagellin Is Required for Host Cell Invasion and Normal Salmonella Pathogenicity Island 1 Expression by Salmonella enterica Serovar Paratyphi A. *Infect. Immun.* **2015**, *83*, 3355–3368. [CrossRef]
9. Ikeda, J.S.; Schmitt, C.K.; Darnell, S.C.; Watson, P.R.; Bispham, J.; Wallis, T.S.; Weinstein, D.L.; Metcalf, E.S.; Adams, P.; O'Connor, C.D.; et al. Flagellar phase variation of Salmonella enterica serovar Typhimurium contributes to virulence in the murine typhoid infection model but does not influence Salmonella-induced enteropathogenesis. *Infect. Immun.* **2001**, *69*, 3021–3030. [CrossRef]
10. Gerlach, R.G.; Jackel, D.; Stecher, B.; Wagner, C.; Lupas, A.; Hardt, W.D.; Hensel, M. Salmonella Pathogenicity Island 4 encodes a giant non-fimbrial adhesin and the cognate type 1 secretion system. *Cell Microbiol.* **2007**, *9*, 1834–1850. [CrossRef]
11. De, R.; Kundu, P.; Swarnakar, S.; Ramamurthy, T.; Chowdhury, A.; Nair, G.B.; Mukhopadhyay, A.K. Antimicrobial activity of curcumin against Helicobacter pylori isolates from India and during infections in mice. *Antimicrob. Agents Chemother.* **2009**, *53*, 1592–1597. [CrossRef] [PubMed]
12. Niamsa, N.; Sittiwet, C. Antibacterial Activity of Curcuma longa Aqueous extract. *J. Pharmacol. Toxicol.* **2009**, *4*, 173–177. [CrossRef]
13. Basniwal, R.K.; Buttar, H.S.; Jain, V.K.; Jain, N. Curcumin nanoparticles: Preparation, characterization, and antimicrobial study. *J. Agric. Food Chem.* **2011**, *59*, 2056–2061. [CrossRef]
14. Liu, C.H.; Huang, H.Y. Antimicrobial Activity of Curcumin-Loaded Myristic Acid Microemulsions against Staphylococcus epidermidis. *Chem. Pharm. Bull.* **2012**, *60*, 1118–1124. [CrossRef]
15. Liu, C.H.; Huang, H.Y. In Vitro Anti-Propionibacterium Activity by Curcumin Containing Vesicle System. *Chem. Pharm. Bull.* **2013**, *61*, 419–425. [CrossRef]
16. Hu, P.; Huang, P.; Chen, M.W. Curcumin reduces Streptococcus mutans biofilm formation by inhibiting sortase A activity. *Arch. Oral Biol.* **2013**, *58*, 1343–1348. [CrossRef]
17. Infante, K.; Chowdhury, R.; Nimmanapalli, R.; Reddy, G. Antimicrobial Activity of Curcumin Against Food-Borne Pathogens. *VRI Bio. Med. Chem.* **2014**, *2*, 12. [CrossRef]
18. Tyagi, P.; Singh, M.; Kumari, H.; Kumari, A.; Mukhopadhyay, K. Bactericidal activity of curcumin I is associated with damaging of bacterial membrane. *PLoS ONE* **2015**, *10*, e0121313. [CrossRef]
19. Gunes, H.; Gulen, D.; Mutlu, R.; Gumus, A.; Tas, T.; Topkaya, A.E. Antibacterial effects of curcumin: An in vitro minimum inhibitory concentration study. *Toxicol. Ind. Health* **2016**, *32*, 246–250. [CrossRef]
20. Teow, S.Y.; Liew, K.; Ali, S.A.; Khoo, A.S.; Peh, S.C. Antibacterial Action of Curcumin against Staphylococcus aureus: A Brief Review. *J. Trop. Med.* **2016**, *2016*, 2853045. [CrossRef]
21. Yun, D.G.; Lee, D.G. Antibacterial activity of curcumin via apoptosis-like response in Escherichia coli. *Appl. Microbiol. Biotechnol.* **2016**, *100*, 5505–5514. [CrossRef]
22. Adamczak, A.; Ozarowski, M.; Karpinski, T.M. Curcumin, a Natural Antimicrobial Agent with Strain-Specific Activity. *Pharmaceuticals* **2020**, *13*, 153. [CrossRef]
23. Marathe, S.A.; Ray, S.; Chakravortty, D. Curcumin increases the pathogenicity of Salmonella enterica serovar Typhimurium in murine model. *PLoS ONE* **2010**, *5*, e11511. [CrossRef] [PubMed]

24. Sifri, C.D.; Begun, J.; Ausubel, F.M. The worm has turned—Microbial virulence modeled in *Caenorhabditis elegans*. *Trends Microbiol.* **2005**, *13*, 119–127. [CrossRef] [PubMed]
25. Couillault, C.; Ewbank, J.J. Diverse bacteria are pathogens of *Caenorhabditis elegans*. *Infect. Immun.* **2002**, *70*, 4705–4707. [CrossRef] [PubMed]
26. Winfield, M.D.; Groisman, E.A. Role of nonhost environments in the lifestyles of Salmonella and *Escherichia coli*. *Appl. Environ. Microbiol.* **2003**, *69*, 3687–3694. [CrossRef]
27. Rangel-Castaneda, I.A.; Carranza-Rosales, P.; Guzman-Delgado, N.E.; Hernandez-Hernandez, J.M.; Gonzalez-Pozos, S.; Perez-Rangel, A.; Castillo-Romero, A. Curcumin Attenuates the Pathogenicity of *Entamoeba histolytica* by Regulating the Expression of Virulence Factors in an Ex-Vivo Model Infection. *Pathogens* **2019**, *8*, 127. [CrossRef]
28. Rudrappa, T.; Bais, H.P. Curcumin, a known phenolic from Curcuma longa, attenuates the virulence of Pseudomonas aeruginosa PAO1 in whole plant and animal pathogenicity models. *J. Agric. Food Chem.* **2008**, *56*, 1955–1962. [CrossRef]
29. Powell, J.R.; Ausubel, F.M. Models of *Caenorhabditis elegans* Infection by Bacterial and Fungal Pathogens. In *Innate Immunity*; Ewbank, J., Vivier, E., Eds.; Humana Press: Totowa, NJ, USA, 2008; pp. 403–427.
30. O'Ryan, M.; Prado, V.; Pickering, L.K. A millennium update on pediatric diarrheal illness in the developing world. *Semin. Pediatr. Infect. Dis.* **2005**, *16*, 125–136. [CrossRef]
31. Bada-Alambedji, R.; Fofana, A.; Seydi, M.; Akakpo, A.J. Antimicrobial resistance of Salmonella isolated from poultry carcasses in Dakar (Senegal). *Braz. J. Microbiol.* **2006**, *37*, 510–515. [CrossRef]
32. Dodds, D.R. Antibiotic resistance: A current epilogue. *Biochem. Pharmacol.* **2017**, *134*, 139–146. [CrossRef] [PubMed]
33. Theuretzbacher, U. Global antimicrobial resistance in Gram-negative pathogens and clinical need. *Curr. Opin. Microbiol.* **2017**, *39*, 106–112. [CrossRef] [PubMed]
34. Berndtson, A.E. Increasing Globalization and the Movement of Antimicrobial Resistance between Countries. *Surg. Infect.* **2020**, *21*, 579–585. [CrossRef]
35. Sasidharan, N.K.; Sreekala, S.R.; Jacob, J.; Nambisan, B. In vitro synergistic effect of curcumin in combination with third generation cephalosporins against bacteria associated with infectious diarrhea. *Biomed. Res. Int.* **2014**, *2014*, 561456. [CrossRef] [PubMed]
36. Leyva-Diaz, A.A.; Hernandez-Patlan, D.; Solis-Cruz, B.; Adhikari, B.; Kwon, Y.M.; Latorre, J.D.; Hernandez-Velasco, X.; Fuente-Martinez, B.; Hargis, B.M.; Lopez-Arellano, R.; et al. Evaluation of curcumin and copper acetate against Salmonella Typhimurium infection, intestinal permeability, and cecal microbiota composition in broiler chickens. *J. Anim. Sci. Biotechnol.* **2021**, *12*, 23. [CrossRef] [PubMed]
37. Udekwu, K.I.; Parrish, N.; Ankomah, P.; Baquero, F.; Levin, B.R. Functional relationship between bacterial cell density and the efficacy of antibiotics. *J. Antimicrob. Chemother.* **2009**, *63*, 745–757. [CrossRef]
38. Bulitta, J.B.; Yang, J.C.; Yohonn, L.; Ly, N.S.; Brown, S.V.; D'Hondt, R.E.; Jusko, W.J.; Forrest, A.; Tsuji, B.T. Attenuation of colistin bactericidal activity by high inoculum of Pseudomonas aeruginosa characterized by a new mechanism-based population pharmacodynamic model. *Antimicrob. Agents Chemother.* **2010**, *54*, 2051–2062. [CrossRef]
39. Li, Z.; Vaziri, H. Treatment of chronic diarrhoea. *Best Pract. Res. Clin. Gastroenterol.* **2012**, *26*, 677–687. [CrossRef]
40. Michael, R.W.; Brown, P.J.C.; Peter, G. Influence of Growth Rate on Susceptibility to Antimicrobial Agents: Modification of the Cell Envelope and Batch and Continuous Culture Studies. *Antimicrob. Agents Chemother.* **1990**, *34*, 1623–1628.
41. Meysman, P.; Sanchez-Rodriguez, A.; Fu, Q.; Marchal, K.; Engelen, K. Expression divergence between *Escherichia coli* and *Salmonella enterica* serovar Typhimurium reflects their lifestyles. *Mol. Biol. Evol.* **2013**, *30*, 1302–1314. [CrossRef]
42. Sargo, C.R.; Campani, G.; Silva, G.G.; Giordano, R.C.; Da Silva, A.J.; Zangirolami, T.C.; Correia, D.M.; Ferreira, E.C.; Rocha, I. Salmonella typhimurium and *Escherichia coli* dissimilarity: Closely related bacteria with distinct metabolic profiles. *Biotechnol. Prog.* **2015**, *31*, 1217–1225. [CrossRef] [PubMed]
43. Pradhan, D.; Devi Negi, V. Stress-induced adaptations in Salmonella: A ground for shaping its pathogenesis. *Microbiol. Res.* **2019**, *229*, 126311. [CrossRef] [PubMed]
44. Wang, H.; Cheng, H.; Wang, F.; Wei, D.; Wang, X. An improved 3-(4,5-dimethylthiazol-2-yl)-2,5-diphenyl tetrazolium bromide (MTT) reduction assay for evaluating the viability of *Escherichia coli* cells. *J. Microbiol. Methods* **2010**, *82*, 330–333. [CrossRef]
45. Wilson, E.; Okuom, M.; Kyes, N.; Mayfield, D.; Wilson, C.; Sabatka, D.; Sandoval, J.; Foote, J.R.; Kangas, M.J.; Holmes, A.E.; et al. Using Fluorescence Intensity of Enhanced Green Fluorescent Protein to Quantify Pseudomonas aeruginosa. *Chemosensors* **2018**, *6*, 21. [CrossRef] [PubMed]
46. Grela, E.; Kozlowska, J.; Grabowiecka, A. Current methodology of MTT assay in bacteria—A review. *Acta Histochem.* **2018**, *120*, 303–311. [CrossRef] [PubMed]
47. Shishodia, S.; Singh, T.; Chaturvedi, M.M. Modulation of transcription factors by curcumin. *Adv. Exp. Med. Biol.* **2007**, *595*, 127–148. [PubMed]
48. Haraga, A.; Ohlson, M.B.; Miller, S.I. Salmonellae interplay with host cells. *Nat. Rev. Microbiol.* **2008**, *6*, 53–66. [CrossRef] [PubMed]
49. Pinaud, L.; Sansonetti, P.J.; Phalipon, A. Host Cell Targeting by Enteropathogenic Bacteria T3SS Effectors. *Trends Microbiol.* **2018**, *26*, 266–283. [CrossRef]
50. Jiao, Y.; Wilkinson, J.T.; Christine Pietsch, E.; Buss, J.L.; Wang, W.; Planalp, R.; Torti, F.M.; Torti, S.V. Iron chelation in the biological activity of curcumin. *Free Radic. Biol. Med.* **2006**, *40*, 1152–1160. [CrossRef]

51. Minear, S.; O'Donnell, A.F.; Ballew, A.; Giaever, G.; Nislow, C.; Stearns, T.; Cyert, M.S. Curcumin inhibits growth of Saccharomyces cerevisiae through iron chelation. *Eukaryot. Cell* **2011**, *10*, 1574–1581. [CrossRef]
52. Sem, X.; Rhen, M. Pathogenicity of Salmonella enterica in Caenorhabditis elegans relies on disseminated oxidative stress in the infected host. *PLoS ONE* **2012**, *7*, e45417. [CrossRef] [PubMed]
53. Cabrera-Diaz, E.; Barbosa-Cardenas, C.M.; Perez-Montano, J.A.; Gonzalez-Aguilar, D.; Pacheco-Gallardo, C.; Barba, J. Occurrence, serotype diversity, and antimicrobial resistance of salmonella in ground beef at retail stores in Jalisco state, Mexico. *J. Food Prot.* **2013**, *76*, 2004–2010. [CrossRef] [PubMed]
54. Galan, J.E.; Ginocchio, C.; Costeas, P. Molecular and functional characterization of the Salmonella invasion gene invA: Homology of InvA to members of a new protein family. *J. Bacteriol.* **1992**, *174*, 4338–4349. [CrossRef] [PubMed]
55. Latasa, C.; Roux, A.; Toledo-Arana, A.; Ghigo, J.M.; Gamazo, C.; Penades, J.R.; Lasa, I. BapA, a large secreted protein required for biofilm formation and host colonization of *Salmonella enterica* serovar Enteritidis. *Mol. Microbiol.* **2005**, *58*, 1322–1339. [CrossRef] [PubMed]
56. Itzia Azucena, R.C.; Jose Roberto, C.L.; Martin, Z.R.; Rafael, C.Z.; Leonardo, H.H.; Gabriela, T.P.; Araceli, C.R. Drug Susceptibility Testing and Synergistic Antibacterial Activity of Curcumin with Antibiotics against Enterotoxigenic *Escherichia coli*. *Antibiotics* **2019**, *8*, 43. [CrossRef] [PubMed]
57. Livak, K.J.; Schmittgen, T.D. Analysis of relative gene expression data using real-time quantitative PCR and the 2(-Delta Delta C(T)) Method. *Methods* **2001**, *25*, 402–408. [CrossRef]
58. Stiernagle, T. *Maintenance of C. elegans*; Caenorhabditis Genetics Center: Minneapolis, MN, USA, 2006; Volume 11.
59. Brenner, S. The Genetics of Caenorhabditis Elegans. *Genetics* **1974**, *77*, 71–94. [CrossRef]
60. Hope, I.A. *C. elegans: A Practical Approach*, 1st ed.; Oxford University Press: Oxford, UK; New York, NY, USA, 1999; Volume 213, p. 304.
61. Amrit, F.R.; Ratnappan, R.; Keith, S.A.; Ghazi, A. The *C. elegans* lifespan assay toolkit. *Methods* **2014**, *68*, 465–475. [CrossRef]
62. Park, H.H.; Jung, Y.; Lee, S.V. Survival assays using *Caenorhabditis elegans*. *Mol. Cells* **2017**, *40*, 90–99. [CrossRef]
63. Kaplan, E.L.; Meier, P. Nonparametric Estimation from Incomplete Observations. *J. Am. Stat. Assoc.* **1958**, *53*, 457–481. [CrossRef]

MDPI AG
Grosspeteranlage 5
4052 Basel
Switzerland
Tel.: +41 61 683 77 34

Antibiotics Editorial Office
E-mail: antibiotics@mdpi.com
www.mdpi.com/journal/antibiotics

www.ingramcontent.com/pod-product-compliance
Lightning Source LLC
Chambersburg PA
CBHW062104220926
51850CB00010B/2886
* 9 7 8 3 7 2 5 8 6 0 7 7 7 *